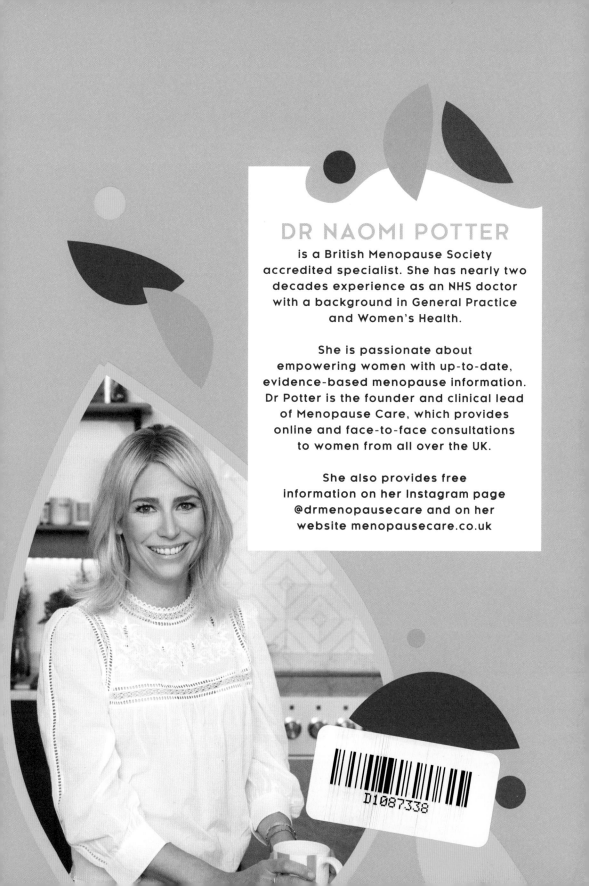

DR NAOMI POTTER

is a British Menopause Society accredited specialist. She has nearly two decades experience as an NHS doctor with a background in General Practice and Women's Health.

She is passionate about empowering women with up-to-date, evidence-based menopause information. Dr Potter is the founder and clinical lead of Menopause Care, which provides online and face-to-face consultations to women from all over the UK.

She also provides free information on her Instagram page @drmenopausecare and on her website menopausecare.co.uk

MENOPAUSING

BY DAVINA McCALL

WITH DR NAOMI POTTER

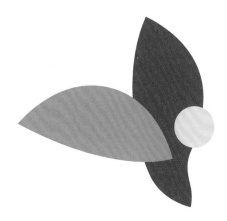

HQ
An imprint of HarperCollinsPublishers Ltd
1 London Bridge Street
London SE1 9GF

First published in Great Britain by HQ, an imprint of HarperCollinsPublishers Ltd 2022
www.harpercollins.co.uk

Text copyright © Davina McCall 2022
Davina McCall asserts the moral right to be identified as the author of this work.
A catalogue record for this book is available from the British Library.

ISBN 9780008517786

Medical expert: Dr Naomi Potter
Editorial Director: Louise McKeever
Designer and illustrator: Imagist
Production: Halema Begum

All author photography © Mark Hayman with the exception of:

p.298 © Davina McCall

Printed and bound in Italy by Rotolito

10 9 8 7 6 5 4 3 2 1

MIX
Paper from responsible sources
FSC www.fsc.org FSC™ C007454

This book is produced from independently certified FSC™ paper to ensure responsible forest management.
For more information visit: www.harpercollins.co.uk/green

While the author of this work has made every effort to ensure that the information contained in this book is as accurate and up-to-date as possible at the time of publication, medical knowledge is constantly changing and the application of it to particular circumstances depends on many factors. Therefore it is recommended that readers always consult a qualified medical specialist for individual advice. This book should not be used as an alternative to seeking specialist medical advice which should be sought before any action is taken. The author and publishers cannot be held responsible for any errors and omissions that may be found in the text, or any actions that may be taken by a reader as a result of any reliance on the information contained in the text which is taken entirely at the reader's own risk.

With huge thanks to all the brilliant contributors and wonderful women who shared their stories.

MENOPAUSING

BY DAVINA McCALL

WITH DR NAOMI POTTER

CONTENTS

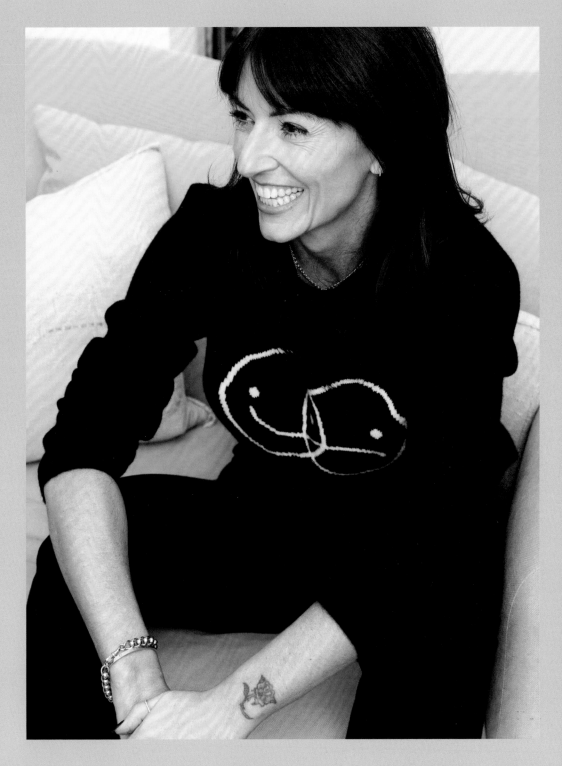

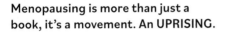

INTRODUCTION:
THIS IS HAPPENING,
PEOPLE ...
MENOPAUSING

Menopausing is more than just a book, it's a movement. An UPRISING.

I don't know about you, but it's quite weird because I can literally pinpoint the first moment when I think my perimenopausal symptoms started.

It's a bit like when a huge, famous event happens, like the death of Princess Diana or Barack Obama becoming President of the United States; I just remember where I was, what I was doing, what I was wearing, what my hair was like ... everything about that moment.

I was forty-four when it started. I remember because it was so WEIRD. The best way I can describe it – and I've heard other women describe it like this, too – is that I just lost something of myself. I changed. I couldn't quite pinpoint how I'd changed, but I'd definitely changed. I didn't feel *myself*.

It was back in 2012 and I was on a Garnier shoot in Prague, working with this amazing director who was asking me to really release my inner beast and be very free with all my movements. I remember feeling more self-conscious and awkward than I would normally and wondering why that was. And each night, when I went to bed – I was there for maybe three nights, in a really nice hotel – the sheets were all lovely and crisp and I'd wake up in the middle of the night and they would be soaking. In the little dent in my neck there'd be a pool of water and I'd be shivering from being cold, because I'd got so hot, then wet, then cold, and I'd have to get up and change the sheets.

I found this particularly horrible because I was a heroin addict a very long time ago, in my early twenties, and the last time I'd sweated like that was when I was using, when I was basically going through cold turkey. I felt SO revolting. With losing all of that sweat and everything, I felt my entire body had turned into a prune, too. My legs were suddenly super-dry when I got out of the shower. My skin was so different; it looked a bit crepe-y and I had to pour moisturiser onto it. I felt as if something changed with my hair, too. And it felt like it had all happened overnight.

Part of me was just thinking, God, maybe I'm ill, maybe there's something going on, maybe I'm out of kilter, maybe I'm not eating properly, maybe I've got some kind of virus? At the time, it didn't cross my mind that the sweats were a symptom of perimenopause.

But what *was* interesting about my perimenopausal symptoms was that they just came and went, a bit like my monthly cycle. It seemed very random.

I didn't have night sweats every night; it was only at certain times during the month. But the other things – the suddenly feeling old, the groaning when I put on my socks, the sensation of my body feeling tired, my mood swings – they felt more constant. It didn't feel like PMS (premenstrual syndrome), it felt like something else. But I didn't know what that was.

One of the worst symptoms was vaginal dryness, which is a miserable, horrible symptom – so much so that I have a whole chapter devoted to it later in the book. I was sore when wiping myself after a wee, with no natural lube to stop the chafing of the loo roll ... TMI? Get used to it. This book is going to be full of it.

Then there was the forgetfulness: my phone was in the fridge, my keys ended up in the bin. This reached really really frightening levels, I forgot EVERYTHING. Words, names, events ... everything!

I think what frightened me most was what happened to my brain, because I work in a job where I wear many different hats for many different TV shows, and I am expected to bring a different kind of energy to each show. And I did a LOT of live television at that time. I remember doing a live TV programme and talking to the contestants, and occasionally looking at them and thinking, *I can't remember your name*. Then thinking to myself, *what was their name?* And I don't know if any of you can relate to this, but it wasn't like something where you just follow the normal neural pathways to remember a memory, when I was looking for this name in my brain, there was nothing there. I literally couldn't think of ANYTHING.

The complete brain fog I put down to sleep deprivation. I thought, well, I'm just not getting enough sleep, that's why I can't think straight. And the way that I was behaving at home was, when I look back at it, unacceptable. I was just always a bit angry. A bit short-tempered, a bit slow, a bit eurgh. I'd lost my love of life.

Anyway ...

I can't just finish that with 'anyway'. And actually, I can't just 'anyway' away that time either. That was quite a long period of my life and I wish I'd known, properly, what symptoms to look out for. I wish that someone that I'd worked with had noticed. I wish I'd learned about it in school so I knew what was coming. I wish that an elder stateswoman had spoken to me about her experience so I could flag up when I was experiencing those things myself.

Because now we know that modern hormone replacement therapy (HRT), modern transdermal HRT (which means it is absorbed through the skin), is largely safe and, in fact, in many ways – and I'll explain this in the book – good for us. I didn't know that, and because of that I lost time in my life. I have spoken to many women in the last year, one of whom had lost nine years of her life fighting to get HRT. Nine years! Then when she got on it, four days later: fine. That's what we've got to stop.

I'm so pleased you're reading this book, and I'm so pleased it's going to be sitting around your house. I'm also really pleased that men and women who come to your house might pick it up and read a bit of it.

After you've read this, pop it on the shelf in your loo. Put it next to the pub jokes book, and make sure that it is available for anyone who fancies flicking through it. *'I'm just going to go and have a quick look at that* Menopausing *book and see if any of these symptoms … '.* Because nobody should have to lose years of their life to menopause, or perimenopause. No one.

Even with all the fantastic menopause books that have been written by great women before me, and all of the programmes that have been made, and all of the women who have appeared on countless TV programmes talking about it, it *still* feels like there is such a hole in our knowledge, and we all know so little about it. And yet it is **absolutely one hundred per cent going to happen to fifty-one per cent of people in this country**. It's crazy.

Around the time when I was really struggling with my symptoms, I was doing lots of live TV, but one show really sticks out. As well as forgetting the stars' names, I was really messing up with my lines. Something weird happened to my eyesight; I just couldn't read the autocue as fluently as I always had done before, and I felt like the words weren't as clear as they usually were, like they were a bit fuzzy when the autocue was spooling forward. It's one thing to make a mistake on a recorded TV programme, but while one fluff you can kind of laugh or joke about on a live TV show, you can't dismiss several.

This lovely lady came up to me afterwards in my dressing room – she's still at ITV now, she's amazing – and she said, 'Are you alright?' And I said, 'Yeah, yeah, I'm fine, don't worry about me. I'm absolutely fine.' And she said, 'Oh good, because I was just checking, because you were uncharacteristically struggling with the autocue and I just wanted to make sure you were ok.' And I was like, 'Yeah, yeah, sorry about that. I'll be fine tomorrow.'

Then she left the room and I just burst into tears. I felt SO bad. I felt SO ashamed, and also scared that I might lose my job, scared that she wouldn't use me again, embarrassed that I'd messed up something that I literally can normally do standing on my head. I was really angry with myself that I'd made these stupid mistakes that I'd never made before. So I was doing one of those angry, sad, frightened cries where you're all of those three things, and I just sat down in a chair and thought, *what is going on?*

Even then I still didn't Google it. Still didn't think about putting two and two together.

But I did talk to my cousin, who is my sort of age, and she said, 'Have you thought it might be the menopause?'. And I was like, no, I hadn't thought that. And she was like, 'Yeah, I'm going through something similar, I think it's the menopause.' Or perimenopause, but we didn't know what we were talking about at that point – it was

like menopause was it, basically, as far as we knew.

Cut to two years later. I'd already called a doctor, worried that I had Alzheimer's. The doctor said, 'You haven't got Alzheimer's, because if you did you wouldn't be calling me to ask me if you had Alzheimer's, one of your relatives would be calling me to ask me if you had it.' She said, 'What you've got, probably, is cognitive overload. You are very stressed out, you've got a lot going on, and you've got three small children; you've just got too much on your plate.'

And that did make me feel better, but I still thought, *God, I just can't think straight. And I'm normally so on it. I'm normally firing on all cylinders, and at the moment I feel like I'm firing on half a cylinder at most.*

I had had moments where I'd sat in the car, having shouted at my kids to try to get them into the car, all three of them, to go to school at the same time. The way that I avoided becoming shouty mum when they were really little was to set my alarm half an hour earlier, and that had worked. But no amount of setting the alarm earlier seemed to be working this time, and I remember sitting in the car one day and saying, 'Look, I'm sorry.' I put my head on the steering wheel and had a little cry. I said, 'This isn't Mummy, I don't know what's happening, but I'm really sorry and let's go to school.' And I just sort

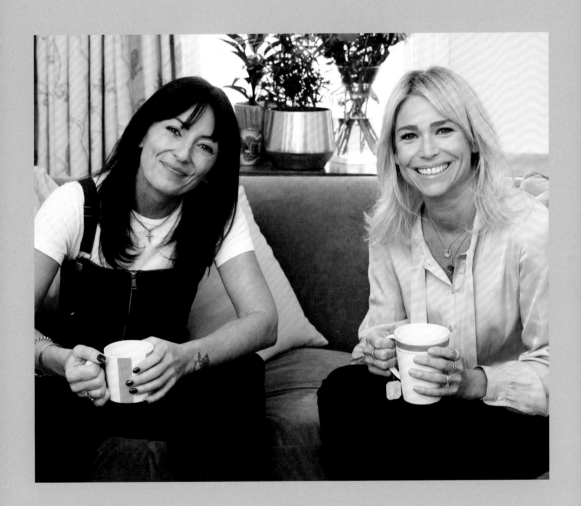

of pretended to be happy all the way to school.

Then in 2014 I did the Sport Relief challenge for charity, and that was CRAZY. Five hundred miles, from Edinburgh to London. On the first day of the challenge, doing hours on a bicycle, my period had started. I wasn't sure when my period was coming or how long it was going to last anymore, as it was all over the place by this point. I had a tampon in (sorry if this is TMI…), and while cycling 130 miles on the first day in the rain the tampon string rubbed and blistered my labia. I had a huge blister and I had to get on a bike every day in soggy cycling shorts for the following seven days – then run a marathon! And, not only that, it was a week when I think because I was very stressed, I got night sweats maybe every other night, and I just wasn't sleeping. I was ABSOLUTELY BROKEN. I mean, new levels of broken. The weather was biblical, I had a period, I was perimenopausal.

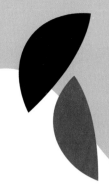

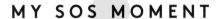

MY SOS MOMENT

In the end, I went back to see my doctor.

I'd previously talked to my GP, who was totally lovely and had said I was probably too young for perimenopause, let's just see how you go.

That did not go down well.

But I've been through some tough times in my life. I'm a recovering addict. I haven't had a drink in thirty years. This wasn't going to break me, right?

I am a wannabe hippy. I had three homebirths, no pain relief ... I did hypnobirthing ... I literally prided myself on being totally badass when it came to pain, or difficult times. I don't like taking over-the-counter pills for headaches, so I was adamant I wasn't going to go down the medical route. I'll up the exercise, I told myself, take a few herbal remedies (black cohosh, anyone?) and drink some herbal teas. My kitchen cupboards resembled a health food store. But nothing worked and I felt worse than ever. I felt a failure.

I was becoming increasingly desperate: at that point if someone had told me that hopping on one leg in the middle of Trafalgar Square, in central London, for three hours would alleviate some of the symptoms, I would have gladly got my hop on.

Look, I adore the NHS and it is always the first place I turn to, but I am also extremely fortunate to have the means to go private if I need to. And by this point, I was seriously worried about my health, so I booked in to see a private doctor. It upsets me writing that, because I know so many of you reading this book won't have that luxury, but this is what I want from this book, to arm you with tools so that you CAN get the support you need from the NHS.

So I went to see a private doctor, who said, 'I think it's the perimenopause, I'm going to send you to a gynaecologist.' And off I went to a gynaecologist.

Anyway, the gynae listened to me run through my symptoms, took one look at me and confirmed I was perimenopausal. OMG!!! THE RELIEF! The tears. I'm not going mad? He was amazing. He was the first health professional who broached the subject of HRT with me, but with the headlines from the early 2000s linking HRT and breast cancer swirling around in my head, I point blank refused to consider it.

He said, 'It is perimenopause, I'm going to put you on oestrogen patches, they're transdermal.' I said, 'I don't want to take them, I'm going to get breast cancer.' He said, 'It's **not** the same anymore.'

I talked to him for a bit, cried for a bit, and then felt like, actually, I would do anything – ANYTHING – to not feel like this anymore. I didn't even care what the slightly increased risks were. In fact, now I know a bit more about the risks, I totally did the right thing, because in my situation, weighing up my life and what I was losing at that time, in terms of the very small additional risk, for me, it was worth it.

My gynae did something that should happen to every single woman as a matter of course, whether you are seeing your local NHS doctor or going private: he actually *listened*. He sat me down, looked at my lifestyle and medical history and step by step took me through all of my individual benefits and potential risk factors of taking HRT. TOTAL game-changer. I wish GPs were able to have longer appointments.

I knew menopause was about hormone levels, but that single consultation opened my eyes to a whole other side of the story. You see, menopause is not just about the short-term impact of our falling hormones – the hot flushes, the brain fog, the mood swings – it's about the long-term risks, too. Risks like osteoporosis, heart disease and there is emerging evidence that it

might even protect against Alzheimer's. This is all super-important, so we'll be exploring this in much more detail in upcoming chapters.

He then told me that in order to be able to take the transdermal HRT patches, which I put on my hips, I also needed to take progesterone, another hormone. He started me off on pills, but the pills made me feel ill, so after a while I went back and asked him if I could have the Mirena coil put in. Interestingly, I'd had the Mirena a long time before, and it hadn't agreed with me. But actually I think that it wasn't that it hadn't agreed with me, I possibly was perimenopausal then, because when I had it put in to counteract the oestrogen in the patch, it was absolutely fine. I've had a Mirena ever since – swapping every five years. And, for me, that's worked really well.

What was amazing was that a few days after I had started this course of HRT, I literally felt the joy come back into my life. And at forty-seven years old, I felt like I was back in a way that I hadn't been for many, many years. I felt SO much better. I felt able to laugh. I felt able to really engage with my children again. I felt bouncy. I felt that I wanted to exercise, and to get up in the morning without a sense of having aged twenty years. My joints weren't hurting. Night sweats were gone. There were lots of ways I didn't realise I'd been feeling bad until I'd taken it, and, suddenly, it was like, 'Oh wow, I really *wasn't* feeling great.' It had a subtle way of bringing me back in ways I didn't realise I needed.

Then came the dark times of deceit, because I spent the next few years trying to pretend to everybody that I wasn't on HRT. Trying to pretend that I'd always been this bubbly and bouncy. That this newfound kind of togetherness that I had, and energy and focus, and ability to read the autocue, was just me feeling great at forty-seven! I lied to friends of mine – I've got a couple of great friends who I love and respect so much, who are homeopaths and naturopaths, and I was so ashamed to admit to them, in particular, that I had gone down the HRT route. I felt that in some way I had failed as a woman, that I was weak. How come other people could soldier on and I couldn't?

So I kept it secret. And I didn't just keep it secret; I lied. If anyone said to me, 'Are you on HRT?', I'd say, 'No.' Then one person would come out of the woodwork and say they were feeling perimenopausal, and I'd secretly whisper, 'Have you talked to anybody about taking HRT?'. At the time, I wouldn't even have suggested going to a GP because I didn't feel like it was on a GP's radar to prescribe any kind of HRT. It had got such a bad reputation, even in the medical world, from all those years ago that I thought it was something you would have to go private and pay for, for the rest of your life. The injustice of it, actually, is rather sickening.

So I lied to my friends. I'd started this secret kind of life as an HRT-taker. A huge change happened when I started to take testosterone as well. Testosterone has been amazing. After being on HRT for a while, I went back to see my gynaecologist and I said, 'I still feel a bit lacklustre, like I don't have much energy, a bit unfocused and bleeeugh.' And he said, 'Ok, well, let's just test your testosterone levels.' He told me, 'Yes, you are low on testosterone, why don't we just put you on that for a bit and see how it goes?'

Testosterone can take a lot longer to take effect in your system, so improvements can take a while. It was not as big a 'ta-da' moment as I had when I took oestrogen, as you're taking such tiny amounts daily; there are limits and you should be within those limits. I was taking what I should for a woman my age. It really, honestly felt – without being a complete cliché –the final piece of the jigsaw. And that's what I call it: it's the final piece of the HRT jigsaw. It is the one hormone that is still incredibly hard to get, and for some reason bathed in shame. We'll talk about that a bit later on in the book…

So that was my journey up to today. About three years ago, I started being honest with my friends, and they were so nice to me. I think at the time they were worried, I think they felt that I was taking an unnecessary risk. But by this point I was so entrenched in feeling fabulous that I wasn't prepared for anybody to talk me out of taking HRT.

My heart goes out to anybody who was on it and then had to stop taking it. I really, honestly, feel for you SO much. But we will talk about, in this book, lots of different ways that you can impact the way that menopause affects you – naturally. So there are ways to control symptoms without HRT, and we'll get to that later. But if somebody tried to talk me out of taking HRT now, I think I'd probably get angry, and I would defend it forever because it has, quite simply, changed my life.

The concept is that some of us who are reading this book could now expect to live till we're a hundred. In the olden days, we didn't have to live for fifty years with dry vaginas and dry skin, aching bones, sore eyes and muscles, electric shocks in our brains and fatigue. We would be dead. But we can't live for another fifty years and have fulfilled lives without sorting out our hormones. Remember, too, that we are not abusing these hormones to become body-builders or superhuman in some way; we are just replacing what we've lost. That is all it is: it's hormone replacement, not extra hormones. And that's really important.

The more we talk about it, the less shameful it is. I want to reframe the way that HRT is viewed by society. I am of the belief that, potentially, women should be offered an appointment at the age of forty-five, 'Would you like to discuss menopause?'. If a woman feels that she, for whatever reason, doesn't want to take HRT, she shouldn't have to. But in terms of saving the NHS money – because of osteoporosis, or heart disease, or potentially caring for somebody with dementia – giving a woman HRT, and giving it to her early, in perimenopause, has many health benefits.

I think we need to reframe the whole way that we look at this. A year's worth of good-quality HRT costs around a hundred times less money than a hip replacement! That's not to mention all those broken bones and all those hospital visits as a result of osteoporosis too. It makes a lot more sense to help prevent these illnesses before they start.

So, here I am. And I did ask myself the question, 'Do I really need to get the message out there to more women? Haven't there been enough books written about this? Isn't the market saturated?' And the more I asked myself that first question, the louder I wanted to shout the answer YES. YES, YES, YES! Because I'm still going on social media every night and being asked questions like, 'Does HRT postpone my menopause? When I stop, won't I just get the menopause then?' No, it doesn't necessarily, and no, you won't necessarily have to stop either. But these are things that we should ALL know. I wanted to make a book that was really simple to use, and clear and simple to read.

We've asked Dr Naomi Potter, who has co-written this with me, to lay out all the sciencey bits and all the facts – because I am clearly not a doctor. I am going to write about my experience as a menopausal woman, and in particular about how all of us can navigate through the next chapter of our lives, so that we all get to live the most fulfilled, happy lives possible.

DR NAOMI'S VIEW

Davina's initial reaction to her symptoms – her confusion and embarrassment – will ring true with so many women.

As women, we are told what to expect when we get our first period. Pregnancy is openly discussed, and quite rightly women get lots of support for this moment in their lives. But when it comes to perimenopause (the time leading up to the menopause, when symptoms begin) and menopause itself, there is a distinct lack of support and openness and many women are left to fend for themselves.

I have seen so many lives affected by a rollercoaster of symptoms. Many women have no idea what is in store for them for the next few months and sometimes even years. And even if they do have an inkling it could be down to the menopause, there is a tendency to want to just 'get through it'.

Davina did what I would urge any woman to do in the same situation: she kept talking, and when initially she was dismissed, she sought another opinion.

Throughout the book, I will be including useful information and key facts. This information will be flagged by pink boxes (as we have here) for ease of use.

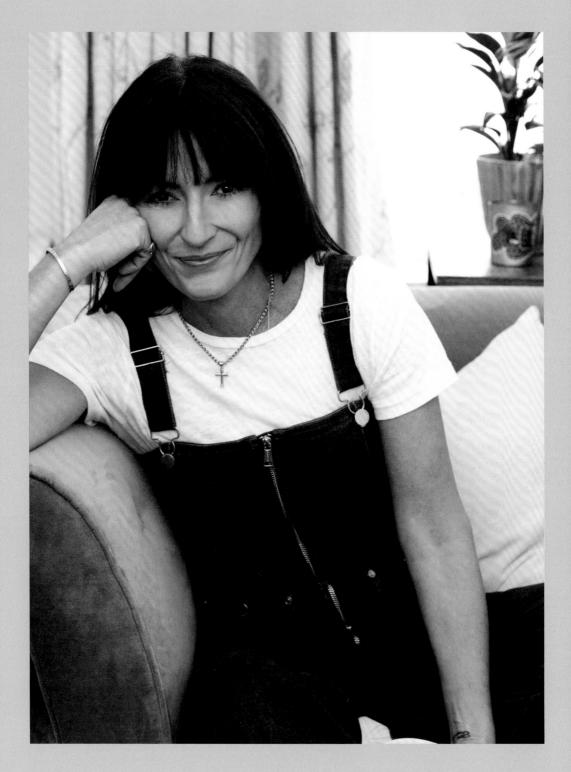

MY MENOPAUSING MISSION

A few years ago I started talking more openly about my menopause. For years I had been aware of the risks of taking HRT, but the discussions I started to have completely re-framed the way I looked at it. And I thought, I have to get this information out there. I can use my reach for good and inform women about their choices.

This is rapidly becoming my life's work. I spend hours every night on social media, sending women I don't know articles or information or guiding them to sites that could help them. But I always feel that this is one woman at a time … I need to do more, and I want to reach more women, which is the whole reason why I've written this book.

These are just a few of the messages I have received on social media:

. . . .

'I'm in the start of this hormone change and I'm really disliking my life … I am lucky to have an amazing partner but I hate the changes happening to my body. This change scares me so much.'

'My doctor needs education ASAP. I'm really struggling and they're trying to get me to try alternative therapies.'

. . . .

'Phone call with doctor to discuss trying HRT. She wants to put me on antidepressants. I'M NOT DEPRESSED!!!!'

Those last three comments pretty much sum up the three humungous problem areas with menopause.

1. THE ATTITUDE PROBLEM

As a society, we have been sweeping menopause under the carpet for generations, harking back to Victorian times when a woman's life expectancy was so short she wouldn't have lived much past the end of her menopause.

Now, the average age of menopause in the UK is fifty-one, and the average life expectancy of a woman is eighty-three years.

Eighty-three years! Do the maths. We have potentially decades of living ahead of us post-menopause, yet this dismissive attitude has stubbornly stuck through the generations.

Remember how your granny or even your mum coped with the menopause? No? Exactly, as they likely never told you or a single soul about it. There's that shame creeping in again, people.

This sort of secrecy persists to the present day, which means that too many women have to resort to guesswork and tons of Googling about their symptoms before they join the dots and make the menopause connection. As Siobhan, an NHS nurse who didn't realise for months she was perimenopausal, so aptly puts it: 'I know it sounds crazy that as a health professional I didn't know what was happening inside my own body, but we just don't talk about it enough.'

2. LACK OF DECENT MENOPAUSE TRAINING

So many stories throughout this book will include 'my doctor refused' or 'my doctor wouldn't/couldn't'. So many of you who shared your experiences spoke of the battles you have had in getting recognition and treatment that I could have filled half this book with these stories alone. And for you reading this now, it may well be that you have had similar experience.

Now, I'm not mad at doctors – it's not their fault (and there are many wonderful enlightened ones out there) – but what I am so, so frustrated about is the woeful training on offer for those very professionals to whom we turn in our time of need. Menopause has not been part of the standard education for GPs or gynaecologists.

Little wonder then that when women go to their GP with a load of symptoms and a whole heap of questions they often don't get the help they so need.

It's time to end the shame and horrific misinformation surrounding menopause.

Who can we trust? Who has the correct information? And how can we get it?

3. HRT MYTHS AND MISINFORMATION

Full disclosure: I'm a big fan of HRT. It's sorted out my symptoms, has given me my quality of life back and is helping to safeguard my future health. End of.

So why did I lie about being on HRT? Because there is such a stigma around it, which stretches back two decades. And that explains why just one in ten women in the UK who would benefit from HRT actually take it.[1]

The crux of the problem lies with data released from the Women's Health Initiative (WHI), a study carried out all the way back in 2002, and the damaging headlines that followed its publication. This study of American women and HRT claimed that HRT increased the risk of developing breast cancer, heart attacks and strokes. But re-analysis of the data has found that the average age of women taking part in the study was sixty-three (remember, the average age of menopause is fifty-one). The fallout was so damaging that women were literally flushing their

---

[1] G.P. Cumming et al. (2015), 'The need to do better – are we still letting our patients down and at what cost?' *Post Reproductive Health*, 21(2), pp.56–62, doi:10.1177/2053369115586122

HRT down the toilet, and numbers of women taking HRT plunged to an all-time low.

Sadly, the negative headlines have stuck, and to this day women find it difficult to access HRT from their doctor, even though it is *the* gold-standard menopause treatment.

All in all, women across the UK have been badly served by society and by science and many feel they have nowhere to turn. They are making enormous life judgements about their health, their future and their sanity, but they aren't in possession of the full facts.

OMG this has to change! And I, along with an army of incredible women, am on a mission to make that change happen.

In 2021, my documentary *Sex, Myths and the Menopause* – which lifted the lid on misinformation surrounding the menopause and examined the

science and fear around hormone replacement therapy – aired on Channel 4. In the days that followed, something really unexpected and amazing happened. I have never ever presented a show that's made so many people want to stop me in the street to talk about it! Not even *Big Brother*. I mean EVERYWHERE I went. On dog walks, in the supermarket, just walking down the street. Some women in tears sharing their stories of feeling invisible, marginalised and patronised. Men and women telling me how much they had enjoyed watching it with their partners and how it had given them a better understanding of what their loved ones were going through. It was totally and beautifully overwhelming.

These encounters and the messages I've received have frequently moved me to tears, because this documentary was deeply personal. These moments have lit a fire in me to make *Menopausing* not just a book, but a mission. An UPRISING.

I'VE GOT YOU

Maybe you are in the throes of the hot flush from hell, or maybe you are buying this book as an investment for the future. **However you came to this book, think of it as your menopause bible. We've got facts, stats, studies, symptoms, sex, relationships and career advice, and plenty of myth-busting, too.**

I'm here to hold your hand and take you through what you need to know.

As I'm no medical expert, I've assembled an incredible team of experts, led by the amazing Dr Naomi, who is a British Menopause Society-accredited menopause specialist, to make sure the advice contained in these pages is practical and based on the latest, bang-up-to-date science.

Dry vagina? Zero sex drive? Hair loss? Want to know if you can start taking HRT for the first time in your sixties? We've got it covered – and much, much more.

And as I've said, what is most important to me is that **every woman will see themselves in the pages of this book**. I just want to thank the amazing women who have agreed to share their own menopause stories.

We'll laugh, we'll cry, we'll get angry, then we'll laugh some more, but most importantly we'll find the answers, together. I want every woman and every man, partner, friend and colleague reading this book to seize the moment for real change.

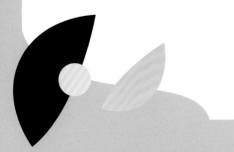

LET'S DO THIS TOGETHER

Here's my three-step guide to getting the most out of this book and starting the Menopausing movement:

1. GET INFORMED:

You owe it to yourself and your health to be as fully informed as possible. We know there is so much noise and misinformation flying around about the menopause, so I have boiled it down to the essential facts. Symptoms, the latest treatments, benefits, risks – you'll find it all in the pages of this book.

2. SPEAK UP:

The time for 'soldiering on' and putting up with menopause symptoms affecting your life, your health and your happiness is over. Now you are informed, you are empowered. Use your knowledge to make the right choices for your health and future – and as a back-up if you are met with resistance.

3. BE AN ALLY:

Menopausing is more than a book. It's a movement. And at the centre of this are honest, open conversations: talking to friends, talking to family, colleagues, jumping on Twitter and busting some myths and offering support to women who might be struggling. We need to share, we need to keep talking ... and *listening*. If you are a health professional or a manager, bring this book into your workplace and hand it around to your colleagues. You don't have to *be* menopausal. You don't have to *be* a woman. These are facts and stories that everyone needs to know.

We've got this.

Ladies, we need to go out there and live our best lives so the next generations don't fear menopause like we did ... or still do. We need to show them that far from drying up and disappearing, we BLOSSOM and flourish. And if that's not you right now ... read this book.

Above all, REMEMBER:

I love you.

It's going to be ok.

I see you.

And I've got your back.

Bookmark this page – or, better still, tear it out and stick it on your fridge, or save it to your phone. Remind yourself daily or whenever you have a wobble and things feel like they are getting too much: together, we've got this.

Are you ready? Then let's get *Menopausing*.

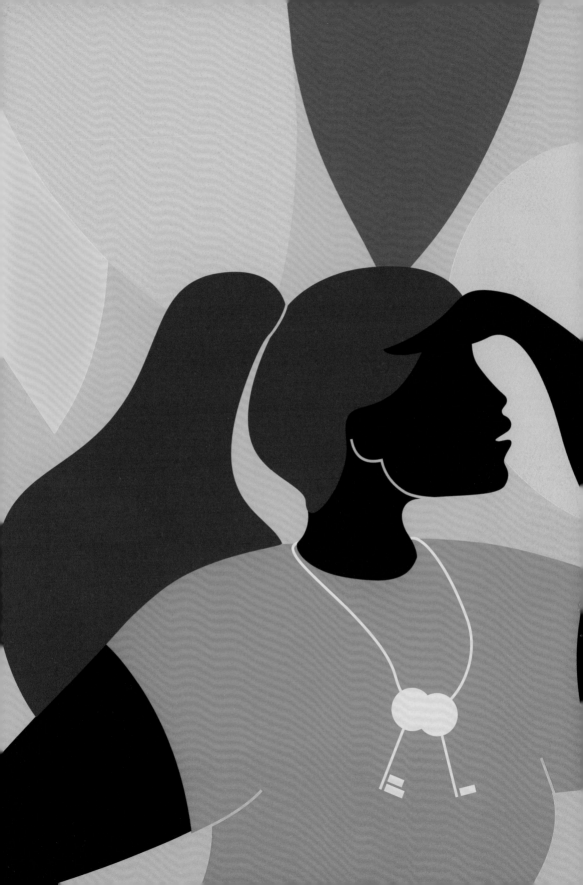

CHAPTER 1

F*** OFF. WHERE ARE MY KEYS?

13 MILLION women in the UK are going through perimenopause or menopause RIGHT NOW

When I first got the symptoms of perimenopause I don't think I've ever felt so alone. I didn't know where to turn, I didn't know who I could reach out to or speak to. So now, if you're reading this book, well, I hope for starters you feel less alone already, because we're all here together. At the back of this book I'm also going to give you an enormous bunch of resources and lovely people to follow on social media who are fantastic menopause warriors and are doing amazing things for women. There is an incredible group of females out there who are offering support, advice and a lovely sense of community.

I feel like this isn't just me writing a book, this is a culmination of all the things that I've learned, all the people that I've met, all the experiences that I've had, or that I've read that you have had, and they've all come together in these pages.

We're all trying to juggle so much stuff – careers, home, kids, dogs, cats and everything in between. I've heard about girls in their twenties coping with early menopause, trans men, non-binary friends, women with cancer, and all unsure of what the right menopause treatments are for them, which is why I *really* felt it was SO important that each and every woman picking up this book should be able to see themselves in these pages. And, I just want to add – when I refer to 'women' in this book, I mean every single person going through the menopause. We are all united in wanting to have a more positive experience.

I wanted to mimic that amazing sense of community that I've found on social media. So I thought I'd put out a shout-out on all my social media accounts, asking any young and old women, trans men – anybody and everybody – to share their stories. Oh. My. God. You were amazing. The response was unbelievable. Within twenty-four hours, hundreds and hundreds of you shared your tales of frustration, fatigue, anger and hope.

It has been depressing and infuriating reading your stories. I don't think I've ever felt so angry about how some of you have suffered. Some of the stories are funny, some are heartbreaking, but you are all badass women trying to make sense of this time that my granny used to call 'the change'. I've actually grown to quite like that name, but I think my favourite expression for it is 'second spring'.

But there's an absolute quagmire of shite we have to wade through before we get to the second spring bit, and that's what I'm here to help you with.

I felt it was important to share some of these stories with you because I want everybody to see a little bit of themselves in this book. I really want you, if you're a bit lost, if you're wondering whether you're menopausal or perimenopausal, I want you to pick up this book, read something and go, 'Oh, I think that's me.'

So, I just want to quickly say, to everyone who responded, thank you so, so, so, so, so much. You are all gorgeous and, above all, you are heard. Your stories, your questions and your experiences are really, I feel, at the heart of this book.

. . . .

'Sore joints, aching legs, crappy skin, candyfloss hair, headaches, itching... the list is endless.' — Sharon

OMG! Where to begin. A couple of years ago – when I first started with hot flushes, in retrospect entering perimenopause – I was so 'I've got this, this isn't gonna be so difficult.' HOW WRONG WAS I?

I don't even know who I am most of the time anymore... Hot flushes – as vile as they are – are the damned easiest of this curse. Brain fog, yeah right, more like complete brain mush. I can't think, I can't speak, I can't process ANYTHING!! I honestly feel like dementia or total shutdown is upon me. I have always been so sharp, so quick-thinking, so eloquent, and now I struggle to even write the simplest of messages without losing the plot (thank God for spellcheck!).

My kids are soooooooooooooooo frustrated, but believe me no one is *more frustrated than me. I don't hear properly – hello tinnitus and visual vertigo (feeling like I've just stepped off the waltzers at a fairground).*

I struggle to translate the words said to me and often take some time to reply. People think I'm ignoring them but it's like being on a transmission delay!!!

Fatigue. Oh my word, such tiredness, every little piece of me and disassociation made (I now realise) so much worse by the antidepressants I have been taking for the past three years!! I'm slowly weaning myself off them. 'Oh hello Sharon, you're back in the room-ish.'

Not to mention the physical changes: the huge belly, sore joints, aching legs, crappy skin, candyfloss hair, headaches, itching... the list is endless.

If I had been around in previous years I would have been sent to an institution. Instead, I've been to see more NHS specialists than most, I've had a whole host of tests – basically working my way down a list of possible causes. Most of them unpleasant, and a little scary at times, and after each one being left feeling I'm imagining each and every symptom when no cause can be found.

Meanwhile, Sharon – the strong, sparkly, social butterfly, successful Sharon – continues to shrivel, continues to hide, continues to despair.

But finally, there was a little acknowledgment from my GP.

Maybe it's my age? Maybe it's the menopause? And we could think about some help for me.

Here are the five things that helped me:
#1 IUD to reduce the bleeding
#2 HRT
#3 Reduce and stop antidepressants
#4 Exercise
#5 YOU, Davina! X

No, Sharon, you did this. You fought on and you managed to get the help that you needed. And I'm sorry, I'm really sorry, and I'm absolutely furious that it took you as long as it did. Love you, Sharon.

. . . .

'I just want to feel whole again.' — Charlotte

This probably started about a year ago. I'm forty-six but feel I'm 106 some days. I look haggard, lack energy, and my self-destructive behaviour has been linked to anxiety.

Where I used to be confident and creative… I am easily distracted, lack focus and concentration… my periods are probably every four months now and very painful.

I just want to feel whole again.

Charlotte's story is heartbreaking. It's short, but I think that we can ALL relate to how she is feeling. It's that wish: *I just want to feel whole again.* Thank you for sharing that, Charlotte.

'Families need to understand that being perimenopausal isn't a choice!' — Saz

I was forty-two and woke up each morning with this deep feeling of anxiety that stayed with me until I eventually fell asleep at night. I was scared and not the person I wanted to be.

My GP said I was burnt out and should sit down more, but with a full-time job, two kids and general running about, taking time out was not high on my agenda! I knew there was more to this than burnout. But who would listen? Who would I turn to?

My body ached, my head ached, my heart ached and my relationship with my husband and kids was suffering, but I tried to be stoic and carry on. Deep down I just wanted to curl up into a ball, cry, and hide from the world. These feelings didn't dissipate, they got worse. Why couldn't I concentrate, why was I grumpy, why did my joints hurt when I was so active, why couldn't I sleep? So many unanswered questions.

After three years of suffering inside and out the doctor agreed to put me on HRT and within ten days I was a different Saz. The Saz that loved to entertain, to meet friends, to have fun and laugh and whoop with joy, and most of all to have time for my gorgeous family, who I'd missed and almost ignored for so long. I suffered in silence for too long. When I look through photos I feel sad to see myself looking vacant, no joy in my eyes, I feel I've missed out on three years of my life.

I'm lucky to live by the sea and be able to go swimming when I can. I would hate for any woman to suffer the way I did, and now I talk about my journey quite openly so others can see how a turbulent time can hopefully be prevented. My family thought I was just grumpy and sad, but families need to understand that being perimenopausal is not something that we choose!

I'm forty-eight now and only wish I had had the support and help sooner and hadn't suffered in silence for so long. Today I laugh more, hug my family and keep the sea close just in case I have a mad moment!!!

Saz, thanks very much for your story. I really identify with looking back at photographs of yourself and remembering how vacant, and kind of empty, and hollow you felt in those photos. I mean, in some of them I'm faking looking happy and I can almost see that I'm faking looking happy. It's hard on our families, but it's really hard because THEY don't know, and actually it's very important for them to read this book too – they don't even have to read the whole thing, just a few of the stories – and it would really help them understand that we are not just being grumpy and sad, we are going through something that is extremely traumatic, and just understanding is so unbelievably helpful. I'm really sorry you didn't get the support and help sooner, but your story will help make sure that other women will.

. . . .

'I'm feeling more like the old me.' — Diane

I was fit as a fiddle and then I turned fifty, and perimenopause hit me like a train. First my eyes started deteriorating, flashing lights and floaters. Of course, at first, I didn't realise it could be down to menopause. Then I was getting terrible sweats – morning, noon and night – palpitations, pins and needles, aching joints.

I had so many issues I went to see the doctor, who said I was very likely just going into menopause. As if it was no big deal!! Straight away he offered me anti-depressants; now thankfully I have never had to need these, so I said to him 'but I'm not depressed.'

Next week I booked up with a female doctor, who was more understanding. She did blood tests and checked my weight and blood pressure. She told me I had different choices. I was hesitant about going on HRT as my mother had breast cancer, but I was willing to try

anything as I literally felt like I was falling apart. I wanted the old me back.

I've been on HRT now for two years. I'm still all over the place some days but I feel 50–60 per cent better than I did before. I weighed up the risks, but I felt I needed to try HRT as my quality of life was crap.

I'm coping ok now. I've got a new job and I'm back out in the world feeling more like the old me.

Oh my goodness, Diane, thanks so much for sharing your story, because it is TERRIFYING how many women get prescribed antidepressants when presenting quite clearly with menopausal symptoms at an age where it is highly likely that you are perimenopausal. I'm so glad that you got the help that you needed. Your story is so important because so many women are going to identify with it. Thank you for sharing.

'It's like menopause doesn't happen to women of colour.' — Zahra

I'm a British Muslim woman, and I'm menopausal. But if you look online or in the pages of newspapers and magazines, you'd think I was the only one. I can't tell you how tired I feel when I see the same old pictures of women trying to cool down with fans, or sitting there with their heads in their hands. The models are always white – where does that leave me and my two sisters?

I'm the eldest girl in my family, so the first among my generation to go through menopause, and I'm determined that my sisters will be more clued up when their time comes.

Zahra, thank you so much for telling us your story, and it was important that we put it in the book, because Muslim women and women of colour are not represented enough in newspapers and magazines in terms of menopause and perimenopause. THANK YOU for speaking out. It is really, really important that ALL women of menopausal age, and trans men, and anybody that goes through perimenopause and menopause should be represented. Your story is important.

. . . .

'I feel as if I've been menopausing forever!' — Sally

I feel as if I've been menopausing for ever, possibly nearing ten years. I naively thought this was something that you went through, and it therefore passed?

The constant hot flushes and chills, day and night and forever putting my handheld fan on and off, the duvet over and off and the window

open and shut. My thermostat is completely broken and just when I think the hot flushes are easing, they come back with a vengeance.

The dry, sore and broken vagina that struggles to do what it was made for … the unimaginable pain! You can't really share that with many people.

The forgetful, muddled fog and calling people by three wrong names till I finally find theirs and sometimes just saying something totally unrelated or not being able to say anything at all!

Stiff aching joints ... is this a symptom too?

The rising anxiety and panic, which has taken me a long time to link to my menopause as I had experienced anxiety periodically over the years, except this is on another level!

Hold on, I'm flushing now – fan out! The familiar sticky, sweaty, and what I call the smell of menopause. Years of poor and no sleep, pleased if I sleep two to three hours at a time.

For years I have thought 'I'm nearly there' or 'it's going to get easier' and 'I can do this'. I've always been reluctant to take HRT as I had a kidney transplant fourteen years ago, and I feel forever blessed and don't want to take anything that may upset my current medication. However, a combination of lockdown, shielding, working from home and forever menopause symptoms accumulating into out-of-control anxiety and panic have resulted in me currently being signed off work, taking anti-anxiety and sleep medication and engaging in talking therapy.

My GP thinks my issues are now more than menopausal and I'm therefore at the point I feel I should at least try taking HRT. Please help me make sense of all of this as I'm still struggling to navigate through it all.

Sally, I think your story particularly breaks my heart, because I can see you've been struggling for so long, and you've been struggling with absolutely terrible symptoms that are *very clearly* perimenopause. I'm amazed that you have managed so well, and pleased that your doctor has suggested HRT. Women with complicated health conditions can be referred to menopause specialists via the NHS, in case anyone reading this is going through something similar.

'I'm a trans man ... why did no one tell me about vaginal atrophy?' — Buck

I transitioned from a woman to a man over twenty years ago.

Unlike some trans men, getting a hysterectomy – or a his-terectomy, as I like to call it – wasn't something I wanted to do, so I chose to keep my vagina, uterus and ovaries. I hated having periods but taking testosterone to suppress the oestrogen in my body took care of that side of things.

After about a decade taking testosterone, I started getting awful cramps, mostly after orgasming. Finding and going to see a gynaecologist as a man with a vagina is an awful experience. I'd have a smear test and be told the cramps would go away by themselves, but I felt fobbed off, like the doctors didn't know what to do with me.

It took a medical emergency when I was living in Mexico to get to the bottom of the problem. One day, after a workout, I passed out cold on the floor.

My then-partner rushed me to the hospital. I had a fever of 101 (39) and it was rising: I'd gone into septic shock. I almost died.

The doctors found that the testosterone I've been taking atrophied my reproductive system: my cervix, uterus and ovaries were fused together, leading to an infection.

Because I still had a vagina and a reproductive system, the lack of oestrogen was causing extreme atrophy.

Those gynaecologists that kept sending me home could have prevented the atrophy with some simple oestrogen cream.

I'd hate for anyone to go through what I did, and that's why I work to spread the message about atrophy in trans males.

Thank you so much, Buck, for your story. I put a shout-out after I realised that I hadn't included trans males and any non-binary friends that wanted to tell us their story, and it hadn't even occurred to me that trans males might go through menopause. I have now learned, and I'm so grateful to you Buck for teaching us what you have gone through as a trans male transitioning. I know how much you do for the trans community, too, so thank you, and thank you for educating me. Lots of love.

'I had just turned forty, but felt like I was 140.' — Jo

My story began in my early thirties. After my first failed IVF I was told I had a very low ovarian reserve. I was told I would find it hard to have a baby and was likely to go through the menopause by my early forties.

Five failed rounds of IVF later, I celebrated my fortieth with my three beautiful, adopted children and began instantly suffering all the classic side-effects: headaches, mood swings, hot flushes, night sweats and a body that felt as though I was 140.

I felt completely alone as none of my friends were experiencing any of these symptoms.

After watching Davina's menopause documentary, I called my GP, and I've been on HRT for about a week now.

I feel better, but I'm still trying to come to terms with my changing body. My body has changed a lot in the last few years, but I have more energy, I ache less and my motivation to move more is helping.

It is good to know I'm not alone.

Oh Jo, it IS good to know that you're not alone, isn't it? And you really, really aren't alone. And I think the other problem is that women before they're forty, if they go to the GP with any kind of perimenopausal symptoms, they can be brushed off as, 'you're just too young.'

But more and more I feel like women are coming forward who are a bit younger, definitely in their early forties – I was forty-four. So thank you so much for sharing your story, Jo.

. . . .

'My perimenopause symptoms were blamed on my disability.' — Jayne

I have a form of muscular dystrophy, which is a genetic condition I have had from birth. It affects my muscles, making me easily fatigued and tired.

I noticed my energy levels dipping more and more in my early 40s. I would have days where I felt absolutely drained, unable to function, more than usual.

At the time I put it down to exhaustion from having a young child and my disability. I had numerous visits to the doctors explaining my symptoms of erratic periods, missed periods, mood swings, tearfulness, fatigue, dizziness, mental fogginess, hot flushes, disturbed sleep. I even asked if it could be the menopause but was told I was too young and instead my disability got blamed for it all.

Now at 46 it has been confirmed I am in fact perimenopausal. I have asked for help with my symptoms, but by the time I got my diagnosis I was an emotional wreck and so the doctor suggested antidepressants were the best course of action for the time being.

I feel quite aggrieved about this because had I been diagnosed earlier and had help sooner with HRT or similar then I wouldn't have had to endure the symptoms for as long as I had, trying to hold my life together and ending up in the state I got to. I feel when you have a disability, yes it can be harder to diagnose conditions which mimic your pre-existing condition but it's also easier for medical professionals to use your condition as a scapegoat rather than look more thoroughly into the causes.

They are also more reluctant to offer HRT due to not always knowing the effect this might have further on a pre-existing condition like mine. When you have a neurological disability, life can be hard enough already but when hormones then start changing these can amplify symptoms and make managing your condition even harder.

I have asked but there isn't any research into muscular dystrophy and the menopause and how it can affect the condition.

Being a woman going through the menopause can be a minefield but there is more and more help being made available. But being a disabled women going through the menopause can be a lonely and harrowing experience due to the lack of research and knowledge about your condition and its interaction with the menopause and the reluctance of professionals to prescribe HRT due to unknown risks.

I am planning to return to the doctors now I'm feeling emotionally stronger to push for more help. I only hope other women in my position get the help they need at the time they need it rather than suffer in silence.

Oh Jayne, this is so important because as you say if you have a disability it just makes getting HRT even harder than IT ALREADY IS.

If your doctor really is not sure, then request a referral.

Jayne, please keep me posted on how you are getting on. x

'Multiple misdiagnoses, career crises and a relationship almost ruined.' — Louise

My menopause story began over four years ago when I started experiencing headaches, vaginal dryness with excruciating itching and irritation, painful period cramps, mood changes, bouts of uncontrollable sadness and sudden forgetfulness.

It was actually my (male) manager who first brought things to my attention. My one-to-ones became therapy. However, my boss's patience was (naturally) running thin, so I Googled symptoms and, voilà! I found the answer: menopause. None of my doctor appointments had combined my symptoms to give an answer. I cried all day once I realised – the relief was overwhelming, it all made sense!

So I made an appointment: no menopause specialist at my surgery, but that was fine, I knew the cause, the treatment was surely HRT, right? The doc said it couldn't be menopause, because I was 'only' forty-three (one year older than my mum was when she went through the menopause), and I should try CBT because it sounded like I had depression.

I took the advice, but things got worse. Home and work were suffering, all I could say was 'I'm not me right now'. So, I returned, saw a different doc, my

husband came too. The doc was newly qualified, he sent me away to see how I felt in a couple of weeks. So, I tried another doc, this time – success!! She gave me HRT patches and the next day was a total transformation!! I was so relieved: I had energy, the brain fog went, sex became appealing again (hubs was pleased!) and I felt like me. I realised it'd been a very long time since I felt that way.

I don't want anyone else to have this experience, I want to help, to end this ignorance and help others.

Louise, your story is brilliant, because you talked about your male manager who brought things to your attention, and I think that it's *really* important that we educate managers, line managers and bosses in the workplace to look out for any of the people that work for them – they need to know the signs of perimenopause.

Sometimes you just need somebody to give you a nudge, or to hear you, or to see you, or to value you enough to say, 'Look, I can see you're not yourself, let's get you back on your feet.'

It was really good to hear your story, Louise, because I think going through menopause in the workplace is really difficult, and some understanding from any colleague, but in particular I would say a male colleague, is extremely welcome. Get a copy of this book given to every male or female manager in an office space.

. . . .

'I haven't let premature ovarian insufficiency hold me back, but it's been an almighty struggle at times.' — Marie

I'm forty-two. I was diagnosed with premature ovarian insufficiency (POI) [menopause under the age of forty] fifteen years ago.

I was in the army at the time and when I was given the news it went something along the lines of:

Dr: You've got premature ovarian insufficiency.

Me: Does that mean I won't be able to have children?

Dr: That's right (no eye contact).

Quite astounding! I've also recently found out that I've been on a third of the dose of oestrogen that I should have been for the past fifteen years. And I hadn't had my hormone levels checked in those fifteen years either. It was no wonder I felt like death warmed up.

And as for libido … pah! I tell you this, not as a whinge, but to support your mission that we need to educate GPs, employers and the general public.

I haven't let POI hold me back, although at times it's been an almighty struggle to keep being the person that I know I am. I was a pharmacist for twenty years but gave that up to focus more on voluntary work. I work voluntarily in overseas disaster relief work, and I am an advocate for a young woman with physical and learning disabilities.

Thank you for listening. Marie xxx

Oh my god, Marie, your story broke my heart. The idea that you have spent fifteen years of your life on not enough oestrogen … it makes me SO angry! I am SO angry on your behalf. You are an amazing woman. Firstly, thank you very much for serving our country in the

army, we really appreciate that.
I am really sorry for what you went
through, and Marie – we heard you.
Thank you again.

'I feel like a shadow of my old self.' — Nadine

I had a partial hysterectomy when I was thirty-seven due to endometriosis, my ovaries were left. Everything was fine until I hit my fifties. Then my world fell apart. I began suffering horrendous anxiety, panic attacks, palpitations, nervousness, light-headedness, tremors, recurring UTIs (urinary tract infections), vaginal dryness, then the auras and migraines started. I battled with my GP for HRT, which after two years I managed to get. It has helped so much with the hot flushes and sleep, but the migraines, anxiety, still plague me, although are not as frequent.

I've been told they will pass but some days they are so debilitating that it feels unbearable; sometimes the headaches can last for days at a time and I have had to take time off work. I have had heart scans, bladder scans, neurology appointments and a brain scan, all I have wanted is for someone to listen to me, I know my body and I know it's

the menopause, but it's such a battle! I just want to feel like me again, confident and happy. At the moment I feel like a shadow of my former self. I used to exercise regularly but now I lack the energy and motivation to do anything. I hate how my body is changing and find it hard to accept this is me. Some days I see glimpses of the old me, then wham! The menopause switch flicks back on.

I'm now nearing fifty-eight and feel that life is passing me by, and I so want to be able to live it rather than just exist.

Nadine, this story really breaks my heart because I don't understand why anyone should have to battle with their GP for HRT when clearly your symptoms are all calling for that. I'm so sorry, and the anxiety is an absolute doozy of a symptom, and so many of us struggle with that. I'm hoping that you will get some answers later on in this book.

'I contemplated suicide – now I am back stronger than before.' — Sally

In 2013, at the age of forty-nine, my periods just stopped; it was like turning off a switch. I then hit the darkest place I had ever been, coupled with the most awful insomnia.

I just couldn't cope, and what made it worse, I was looking for a reason WHY.

My GP diagnosed depression, I was signed off work and put on antidepressants. I sat up night after night, with the dog for company, whilst my husband slept. We are dairy farmers: he works hard, and the business had to go on regardless of me. In the early hours was the worst, I rang the Samaritans regularly, I didn't want to go on, I hadn't the strength, everyone would be better without me. I contemplated suicide. I hated the person I had become. I had also gained loads of weight, which didn't help, I saw a fat useless lump.

But I had good friends, one of whom got me to join the gym. I found it hard to go but forced myself. I liked the treadmill, this led to short jogs around home, where I was seen by the leader of our local running club. 'Join the Couch to 5K, it will help, you know,' they said.

So I started, even though I had never run before, going while knackered without

sleep, I just kept going. No other choice, I was fast running out of options. At this time, I found myself going for counselling, for me it made things worse, again looking for answers. I went through two counsellors, until I actually found a lady who made sense. To this day I still book the odd catch up (as a personal MOT). I see her now as a friend and her walking therapy is a breath of fresh air.

This, along with running, helped. Soon I was running 5K and starting to believe in myself. It was baby steps. By 2018, I had lost two stone and run my first half marathon, and this is from a lady who 'didn't run'. My husband and daughters and grandson were at the finish to cheer me on. I am still running three times a week and go to a gym in a garage on a local farm. We train outside in the garden. It's a lovely bunch of ladies who support each other, we work hard and laugh loads. I very seldom go to the doctors now, and counselling occasionally.

I am proud that I did this myself. The antidepressants are less than half a tablet now.

And the old Sally? Well, she is back stronger and better than before.

Sally, thank you SO much for telling us your story. I'm really sorry that life got so dark for you, but I'm really grateful that you have told us the way that you got through it with exercise. Because for women who don't want to take HRT, or who can't take HRT, this is a really, really important lesson. We're going to be talking a lot about exercise and how crucial it is in terms of mental health, physical strength and bone strength later on in the book, but your story is a fantastic example of that. You should be proud of yourself. You. Are. Badass.

. . . . . .

'Help! Menopause is a minefield!' — Lou

I was so confident that I had escaped the menopause 'Thing'.

If you'd have asked me two years ago, aged fifty-five, I would have said something like 'don't know what all the fuss is about', or 'guess I'm just lucky but I didn't really get any of those things.'

Then I started feeling like every morning was an effort to get out of bed, feeling like an old lady, with stiff, heavy legs. I didn't start to feel awake till lunchtime and by three in the afternoon I'd be thinking I could really just lie down right now and sleep.

My boobs ballooned and my hips too. My belly, which was always pretty flat, became constantly bloated. Two years on trying various exercise routines and diets with no great effect I am now suffering from an incredibly painful legs which keeps me awake all night some nights.

I've seen doctors and had physio sessions but no change. I have finally concluded after lots of reading and research, my ailments – now a growing list – can very well be down to menopause.

That said I'm no closer to a solution because it's a minefield nobody seems to understand.

Lou, it's funny isn't it, how sometimes you can be a bit kind of smug and sort of think … it's really not that bad, I'm absolutely fine, I've got through the perimenopause thing, no problem … and then it hits you like a freight train. Keep going to see doctors, keep asking for advice, maybe ask to go and see a menopause specialist (ask your doctor). But I just want to send you SO much love and thank you for sharing your story.

CHAPTER 2

KNOWLEDGE IS POWER: PERIMENOPAUSE AND MENOPAUSE EXPLAINED

'Can I go on HRT if I'm still having PERIODS?'

'Do I need TESTS?'

'It's not menopause – I haven't had any HOT FLUSHES'

'What's happening to me????'

I think, like a lot of you out there, menopause just wasn't a topic of conversation for the dinner table when I was growing up. Nobody talked about it. Our elders didn't talk to us about it. My grandmother would refer to 'the change', but never to *me* – I would hear it in the background with her friends, or whatever. She never would talk about it to *me*, because I was a little girl when I lived with her.

So perimenopause literally crept up on me like some evil gremlin, and I was not equipped or confident in knowing WHAT THE HELL to do about it.

I reached out; I reached out to my cousin, and I spoke to a few friends. I don't really have many friends that I'm super-close to in the business who are older than me, so I didn't really have anybody to talk to. Seeing people in the public eye – people like Lorraine Kelly and Liz Earle – that's been really helpful, and they've made me feel safer about opening up about my own menopause.

And obviously, recently, Michelle Obama – fucking legend, I love that woman! She talked about having hot flushes while riding in the Presidential helicopter. I mean, that is really, really big! Michelle Obama – that woman is ON IT, and if she's on it, there's hope for me. If you can be the First Lady, look that smoking-hot, write books, do charity work and sit down next to world dignitaries night after night, then I've got this!

But right now there's a new wave of women who really are banging the Menopausing drum, and who are prepared to talk really openly and honestly about their experiences. And if they can discuss it, SO CAN WE.

Talking about it is *so important*, because the stigma attached to discussing the menopause has run for centuries. It runs deep in the female psyche. And I want our husbands, brothers, fathers, partners, to be able to talk about the menopause without giggling. It's NOT FUCKING FUNNY.

Let's break down that stigma that it's just part of something that happens. It's something that some of us need a bit of support with at times, it's something that we need to talk about. We certainly need to share it with other women, and we need to share it with young girls. And with young boys, too. Everybody needs to know about it, because it's definitely going to happen, and it's going to happen to someone you know, if it's not already happening to you.

We've really got to fly the flag for all women out there. I want to show you it's going to be ok, but together we need to learn the basics so we can inform ourselves, and – really importantly – each other. Hormones. Oestrogen. Progesterone. Periods. No more periods. Do I need blood tests? Am I 'in' menopause? What IS menopause? Am I out the other side?

When you look online, it is an absolute quagmire of confusion and misinformation. And the real problem with looking online is that often there are no dates next to the piece of medical information that you're reading. So you might be reading a piece about a specific issue that you're facing with your perimenopause or your menopause, but this information could be five, six years old.

And I'm telling you that with all the *amazing* inroads that doctors and scientists are making with regards to perimenopause and menopause right now, anything you read that's older than two or three years could be out of date.

So many things are changing. The guidelines are changing ALL the time. (The only thing that's bloody not been changing is the misinformation on the leaflets inside the HRT boxes, but we're hoping that's going to happen at least by the time this book comes out.)

So, we need answers. You might have a bit of an inkling that your menopause train is already in motion, or you might just want to prepare yourself for what's coming down the track. Whatever your reasoning, it's time to activate step one of the *Menopausing* Mission.

Now, I know that if I had been better informed, I think I would have been more comfortable talking about my experiences and getting help sooner; if I had known that it's not embarrassing

and it's something that can be fixed so easily. Actually, I'm lying, it's not that easy at all ... but *it is* something that can get fixed and hopefully this book will make it easier. If I'd known that, I would have got help sooner, and I would not have gone through those three or four dark years.

Like many people have said in the stories at the beginning of this book, we're never going to get those years back. And this is terrible. We should help other women to not lose those years when we should be having the time of our lives!

We talk about menopause in my house a lot, as you can imagine, around the dinner table. And it's not just with Holly and Tilly, my girls, but with my son Chester, too. They all know what the perimenopause is, the menopause, and they know about symptoms, they know about hormones, and – most importantly – they know that there's no shame attached to it.

So, with the help of the lovely Dr Naomi, I have put together a bit of a masterclass that cuts through the misinformation and takes you straight to the essentials. The who, the what and the why of the perimenopause and menopause. So I am basically your *much* wittier version of Google.

The answers that you need right now
are to questions about:

1.   Hormones

2.   Perimenopause

3.   Menopause

4.   Getting a diagnosis

5.   Long-term health risks you need
     to be aware of

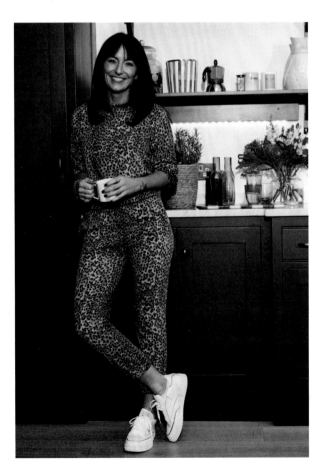

GRAB YOUR LAB COAT, IT'S TIME FOR A BIOLOGY LESSON

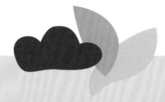

DR NAOMI'S VIEW

In my years caring for patients, I know one thing is for certain: there is no such thing as a textbook menopause. For some patients the symptoms can hit seemingly overnight, while for others it is more of a gradual realisation that something isn't quite 'right'.

One of the main questions I will hear from patients during their first appointment with me is, why? Why am I feeling like this, why is this happening to me?

To address the why questions, the first place to start is with our hormones – what they are, how they work and why they are so important.

WHAT ARE HORMONES AND WHY WE DO WE RELY ON THEM?

Hormones are our body's chemical messengers, which are sent off into the bloodstream to our tissues and organs.

Hormones are essential: they have many functions – from regulating mood, to growth, metabolism, sexual health and reproduction. It is a matter of balance: having too much, or too little, of a hormone can lead to all sorts of symptoms and potential problems.

The main hormones we'll be referring to are oestrogen and progesterone.

Oestrogen is mainly produced in the ovaries. These are two organs, one of which releases an egg each month. There are oestrogen receptors on cells throughout the body. Oestrogen keeps our bodies in tip-top condition, from helping to regulate our menstrual cycle to boosting our mood and memory, strengthening our bones and protecting our heart.

Progesterone helps regulate our menstrual cycle, preparing the body for conception, and keeping our bodies happy and healthy during pregnancy.

Another hormone we'll be talking about a lot is testosterone. It can be the missing piece of the puzzle when it comes to HRT. Testosterone isn't just for men – it helps to regulate our mood, sex drive, strength, stamina and power. It does decline in women during the menopause, but the decrease can be unpredictable.

SO, WHAT DO THESE HORMONES HAVE TO DO WITH PERIMENOPAUSE AND MENOPAUSE?

The definition of menopause is when you haven't had a period for twelve consecutive months. This can be a bumpy road: hormones can fluctuate for several years before you get to the menopause, during a transition phase known as perimenopause. It's these hormone fluctuations and then the subsequent loss that causes symptoms during perimenopause and menopause.

PERIMENOPAUSE EXPLAINED

Confused by what symptoms to look out for? Gone to see your GP only to be told your bloods are 'normal'? Or maybe you've been told you are simply 'too young' to be perimenopausal?

For a long time, there has been a misconception that symptoms only start with menopause. But more often than not, this isn't the case. Symptoms can begin years before your periods stop completely, and they can be super-debilitating. There is so much confusion and misinformation around perimenopause that I would dearly love to be able to write you one of my wonderful lists on what to expect, and when, so you can tick off symptoms like a to-do list.

Sadly the perimenopause isn't like that – because it is a transition phase, it's a time of fluctuations in hormones and turbulence. The ovaries are starting to wind down hormone production but hormone levels can yo-yo, meaning you may experience these symptoms for months, only for them to resolve and you feel 'fine' again. BUT even if I can't give you a neat list, what I can do is give you facts to help you to listen to your body and act if and when you need to.

WHEN DOES PERIMENOPAUSE HAPPEN?

Lots of women who contact me will be, like I was, in their early to mid-forties when they first start showing signs of perimenopause. But please don't ever think you are 'too young' to be perimenopausal. We're all unique and there is no such thing as an 'average' perimenopause and menopause. Everyone's experience will be different – for some, perimenopause will start much earlier, or the menopause can happen overnight due to a health condition or treatment. If you're going through an early menopause right now, skip to chapter 4, I've got you covered.

HOW TO TELL IF YOU ARE PERIMENOPAUSAL (HINT: IT'S NOT JUST ABOUT YOUR PERIODS)

Dr Naomi is such a force for good and an incredible font of knowledge in the menopause world. She does these amazing Instagram lives that just explain perimenopause and menopause in such simple, straightforward terms.

One of the first times I chatted with Dr Naomi, she referred to the perimenopause as the 'master of disguise'. It's such a brilliant way of looking at it, because it can manifest itself in practically every way. So many symptoms can be because of perimenopause.

Lots of women I talk to will say it all starts with a hunch, a feeling, or a slow realisation that something is changing. Maybe you have spotted a symptom that wasn't there a few weeks or months ago, but usually you can't put your finger on it.

Because menopause centres around the end of periods, a lot of women will tend to focus on their periods stopping altogether. But in reality, periods stopping is one of the last symptoms to occur, and you can have regular periods for years in perimenopause. My periods were definitely different but I didn't really pay much attention. Looking back, it's because I didn't really know what perimenopause was, and I ruled out menopause because I thought I was too young. It probably took me about a year before I started to join the dots and realise everything was connected.

It is completely normal for periods to change in perimenopause. They can become frequent, less frequent, longer, shorter, lighter and heavier. If they are persistently heavier, especially if you are over forty-five, extra investigations may be needed to check the lining of your uterus.

The focus on periods can mean that other symptoms – such as itchy skin, vaginal symptoms, hair loss, low libido and many more – can start years earlier but can get missed.

'All the things I loved doing became meaningless.' — Fiona

Fiona, who is going through perimenopause, describes 'staring at my fifty-year-old self in the bathroom mirror watching my youth fade away.' I really related to this.

To say the last few years have been a rollercoaster of emotions and mood swings would be an understatement. It is hard to explain to others what you are going through when you don't fully understand it yourself. It's not like you suddenly wake up feeling different – the changes are so subtle at first that it's easy to dismiss them. For me, it was a gradual loss of my joy, my enthusiasm, my energy and passion for life. Not only did I feel I was losing myself, but my mind too. Although I'd always suffered with anxiety, it was now through the roof. All the things I loved doing became meaningless because the happy feelings they used to trigger were missing. It was like all the colour had been drained from my life and I didn't know how to get it back – how to reconnect with my true self again. Where was I? All I could see was an imposter – an angry, scared and irritable woman who couldn't remember if she'd brushed her teeth or put on deodorant that morning.

Often anxiety and a bit of low mood are the first symptoms and that anxiety can be very subtle but really debilitating. Somebody who is quite confident and outgoing in their life might suddenly start to feel a bit nervous about driving at night, or being in social situations when they never were before. These things are very undermining to your confidence, and in turn can make you feel quite sad, with the hormones compounding that.

It quickly starts this really negative Catch-22, where you're in a downwards spiral, and it's your hormones. But I think people attribute it often to your age, or getting older, as if it's just a getting-older thing, but actually it is your hormones.

SO, <u>ARE</u> THERE ANY EARLY SIGNS YOU MIGHT BE APPROACHING PERIMENOPAUSE?

When I was still having periods, I was regular as clockwork. I was really lucky – twenty-eight days, bosh! I was on the contraceptive pill but, oh my God, PMT was terrible. For about a week, I would be a bit tetchy, a bit moody, a bit weepy. My boobs would hurt, I'd feel bloated, I'd feel revolting. And then on the first day of my period: miles better.

Loads of you who shared your stories identified with that. I heard about that a lot. About three-quarters of women will suffer from PMS, and if you experience worsening PMS - when it is really intense – this can be a sign of perimenopause.

'No one ever talks about this part of life.' — Johanna

Johanna was told she was perimenopausal in her early forties, after years of struggling with PMS:

I spent years hating everyone at certain times of the month and had bad night sweats (though these stopped about two years in), painful breasts, but clockwork periods. Then came about a year of incredibly heavy periods but still fairly regular, with the odd one missed. Then, when I was forty-seven, they stopped. Completely. To be replaced by periodic hot flushes, in the evening, at about 9pm! Not every night, and not every week, but every few weeks. Almost cyclical. Then after about eighteen months, they stopped. However, aching joints have started, and weight gain.

I'm assuming I'm well into the menopause now? At fifty-one I'm still not sure what's what. No one ever talks about this part of life. It's confusing and seems to vary so much from person to person.

Well, I am writing this book for you, Johanna. This is where you will find the answers.

If you have PMS, your body is sensitive to the hormonal changes that take place during the menstrual cycle. Oestrogen levels peak in the middle of your cycle and are at their lowest during your period. Levels of progesterone – the hormone that prepares the body for a potential pregnancy – are highest in the second half of the cycle, the time between when you ovulate and when your period starts. PMS can get worse during the perimenopause and can be one of the heralding symptoms.

HOW LONG WILL PERIMENOPAUSE LAST?

This can vary – it might be a couple of months, or it can go on for years. On average, though, perimenopause lasts for about four to eight years.

DO I HAVE TO WAIT UNTIL MY PERIODS STOP BEFORE STARTING TREATMENT?

This is definitely not the case, you can start HRT during the perimenopause and it can greatly relieve your symptoms. If you are still having periods you will need to use sequential HRT, which we will discuss in more detail later in the book.

This really annoys me, that women often get told by people that they can't have HRT or other treatments if they're still having periods. That's codswallop! **NO! NO NO NO!** I'm telling you now there's absolutely no reason to wait, because you can get the benefit of treatment way before that.

I started HRT during perimenopause, and it saved my bacon. Honestly, I'm not sure I would still have a job now if I hadn't, and I definitely wouldn't have been able to even generally keep my shit together had it not been for replacing those hormones.

I am a huge advocate for freedom of choice, so you have to weigh up the options for you. And that's what this book is all about. We are going to tell you everything you need to know so you can make an informed decision about your own body.

Perimenopause can go on for several years, and during that time you might be at the top of your game, or you might need energy to keep up with your growing kids, and, sadly, maybe look after your ageing parents, too. And all of this can be massively affected by these terrible, rollercoaster hormones. So, starting treatment during this nightmare time can help you get on with living your life to the full.

I often hear from women on social media that they have been to their doctor and had a blood test, then they've been told that their hormones are absolutely fine. Here Dr Naomi explains why this is not necessarily the case.

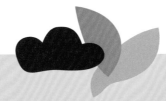

DR NAOMI EXPLAINS

It can be confusing to know when the menopause has begun and when the perimenopause turns into the menopause, but the menopause is when you haven't had a period for twelve consecutive months. However symptoms can begin earlier. The average age of menopause in the UK is fifty-one.

WHEN SHOULD I SEE A DOCTOR?

This is up to you, but if struggling, you are entitled to help. Unsure whether to make an appointment? Ask yourself:

→ Are your symptoms affecting your life, relationships or work?

→ Are symptoms worrying you?

→ Do you need advice on what to do?

→ Do you need to get a second opinion? This might not be your first visit: if something is not right, see another doctor.

→ Have you tried HRT but it hasn't worked, or have you experienced negative side-effects?

If the answer to any of these questions is yes, it is worth visiting your doctor.

GETTING A DIAGNOSIS

If you're not on any kind of hormones, actually finding out if you're perimenopausal or not by taking a blood test is really difficult, because your hormones are going to be all over the shop. They're going to be up and down one day, really on the floor the next, then absolutely fine another day.

It is often assumed that a blood test is the definitive way to diagnose perimenopause, but in most cases a diagnosis can – and should – be made following a discussion with your doctor, taking into account your age and your symptoms. The National Institute for Health and Care Excellence (NICE) menopause guidelines say that at forty-five if a woman is presenting with symptoms typical of the menopause, the first line of treatment should be a treatment of HRT.

If you're over forty-five, as I've said, and you've got typical perimenopause or menopause symptoms, there is therefore no need for you to have blood tests unless your doctor suspects that something else might be causing your symptoms. If you are under forty-five, your doctor will probably want to carry out investigations to look for an underlying cause and confirm perimenopause if that is their suspicion.

These include the following tests:

→ Follicle stimulating hormone (FSH) test: This hormone essentially stimulates the ovaries, and a raised FSH level can indicate you are perimenopausal or menopausal because your brain is having to work harder to get your ovaries to respond. However, the test can be unreliable because hormone levels fluctuate and should be repeated after a confirming diagnosis. If you're on the combined contraceptive pill, this can also affect the accuracy of the result.

→ Oestradiol test: Oestradiol is a type of oestrogen produced in the ovaries. Low levels can indicate the perimenopause or menopause, but because hormone levels vary this can be unreliable.

Other tests might also be carried out to rule out other causes of your symptoms. These include:

→ Full blood count (FBC): This is a very common blood test that checks the type and numbers of cells in your blood. It can give a good picture of your overall health and pick up potential problems such as infection, inflammation or anaemia.

→ Liver function test.

→ Thyroid function test: The thyroid is a gland in the neck which produces hormones that help to regulate body functions such as heart rate and body temperature. When your thyroid produces too much or too little hormones, this can result in symptoms such as changes to periods, mood changes, weight changes, tiredness and difficulty with temperature regulation.

→ Vitamin D test: a deficiency can present with similar symptoms as the menopause.

→ Urine analysis for bacteria, to check if you might have an infection.

BLOOD TESTS

Blood tests can be helpful when you are established on HRT to check absorption, but at the diagnosis stage these aren't normally needed if you are over forty-five. Expensive, complicated investigations are not usually needed either. These include saliva tests, dried urine tests, hair sampling and DNA sampling. These are not in the British Menopause Society guidelines and are not performed by British Menopause Society-accredited specialists.

So, to be absolutely clear:

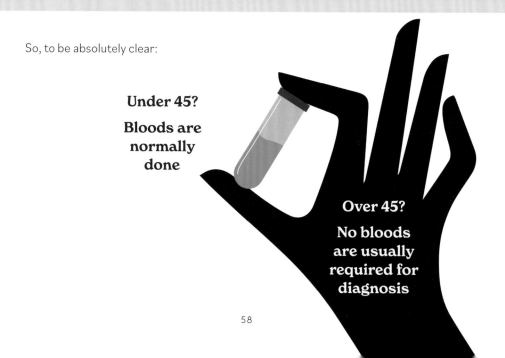

Under 45?

Bloods are normally done

Over 45?

No bloods are usually required for diagnosis

WHY WE HAVE TO GET
THE WORD OUT AND
SHARE OUR STORY

'I talk very openly about any part of my journey ... I feel stronger for it.' — Kirsty

When I first read Kirsty's story, it leapt off the page. I love the opening line:

Perimenopause simmered for about four years before slapping me in the chops with a wet fish overnight.

For the past four years I have been completely open about my experience, shouting it from the rooftops to anyone who would listen, and determined to help people.

I talk very openly about any part of my journey ... I feel stronger for it. It's not going to get me down. I laugh about it and if I have a brain fog moment, everyone knows cos I tell 'em.

Oh my God, I SO identified with Kirsty's story. She described all the 'classic' symptoms: her confidence was shot, she had brain fog, going from having an 'amazing memory' before the menopause to barely being able to remember her name some days.

She was so worried she asked her doctor for a brain scan and was willing to go private for it. Stress and anxiety meant she would end up in floods of tears and be sent home.

Four years on, she's on HRT, and after a few adjustments she's back on top, where she belongs.

Wet fish analogy aside, what really struck me about Kirsty's story was her determination to share her experiences to help others. We all need to be more Kirsty. This is happening, people, we have to share, we have to learn and we have to listen to help each other through.

LONG-TERM HEALTH IMPLICATIONS YOU NEED TO BE AWARE OF

The symptoms of perimenopause and menopause can be very tough, but declining hormone levels can also have health implications long term.

The symptoms of perimenopause and menopause can be improved by HRT. But taking HRT can also reduce the risk of osteoporosis, the frequency of urinary tract infections and the risk of cardiovascular disease. There is also emerging evidence it may protect against dementia, Alzheimer's and other neurological conditions.[1]

OSTEOPOROSIS

Osteoporosis is a condition that makes our bones more prone to fractures. About three million people in the UK are thought to suffer from osteoporosis, but the condition is a lot more common in women.[2]

Our bones are at their strongest in early adulthood, but we all start to lose bone density from our mid-thirties onwards. Oestrogen helps to maintain our bone structure and strength. The loss of oestrogen after menopause can accelerate the loss of bone density and put you at risk of osteoporosis. Osteoporosis isn't a painful condition, which means it often only gets diagnosed after a fracture which can be from something as minor as a bump or fall. Taking HRT can improve bone density.[2]

CARDIOVASCULAR DISEASE

Heart disease is the number one killer of women in the UK. In fact, coronary heart disease kills more than twice as many women as breast cancer.[3]

Cardiovascular disease (CVD) refers to conditions affecting the heart or blood

---

[1] Yu Jin Kim & Maira Soto et al. (2022) 'Association between menopausal hormone therapy and risk of neurodegenerative diseases' Center for Innovation in Brain Science, University of Arizona, Tucson

[2] Bowring CE, Francis RM. Royal Osteoporosis Society's Position Statement on hormone replacement therapy in the prevention and treatment of osteoporosis. Menopause International 2011;17:63_65.

[3] British Heart Foundation (2022), 'UK Factsheet', https://www.bhf.org.uk/-/media/files/research/heart-statistics/bhf-cvd-statistics---uk-factsheet.pdf

vessels, including heart disease, angina, heart attack, high blood pressure, stroke and vascular dementia.

CVD affects around seven million people in the UK, and you are more at risk if you have diabetes or a family history of heart disease, and if you are a smoker.

Declining oestrogen during and after menopause increases the risk of CVD. Oestrogen helps to keep the arteries (which carry blood away from the heart to other parts of the body) smooth and flexible. Once oestrogen declines, your arteries are more prone to developing a lining of fatty plaque, which narrows the arteries and makes you more likely to have a heart attack or stroke. Oestrogen also helps to regulate cholesterol levels and body fat distribution – too much fat around your mid-section also increases the risk of CVD.

DEMENTIA

Worldwide, women with dementia outnumber men two to one.[4] The exact reason behind this is not yet known.

We do understand that oestrogen protects against vascular disease, and one of the causes of dementia is vascular dementia. It is therefore logical to assume that HRT can prevent vascular dementia.

There are a number of different types of dementia and there is emerging evidence that HRT may well protect against those as well, but further research is necessary.

These statistics completely blew my mind. My dad had Alzheimer's, and this is an area I cannot believe that we are not literally piling money into researching further.

---

[4] Alzheimer's Society (2018), 'Why is dementia different for women?', www.alzheimers.org.uk/blog/why-dementia-different-women

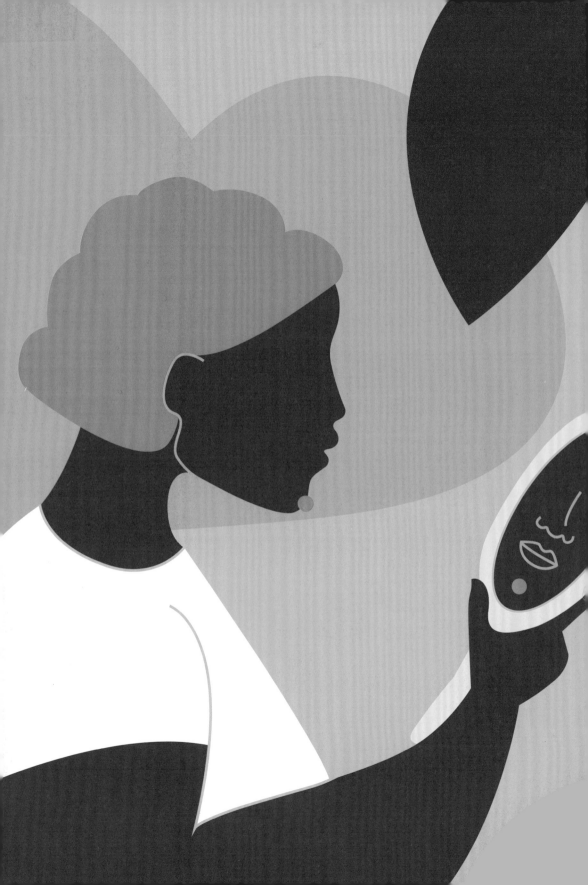

CHAPTER 3

FROM DRY VAG TO ZITS: SIGNS YOU MIGHT BE PERIMENOPAUSAL OR MENOPAUSAL

HOT flushes
COLD flushes
Anxiety
RAGE
Bleeding gums
Forgetfulness
Electric SHOCKS
(I know, right – WHAT?!)

When oestrogen levels fall, the gloves are OFF. Literally, it just attacks every part of your mind and body. I had my own whopper list of really horrible symptoms, but I feel like the brain fog and forgetfulness were the most scary – and debilitating – of these. I think probably this is because of my family history of Alzheimer's and the unfounded fear it could be Alzheimer's.

It's interesting – my dad and I were very, very similar; I was always a proper daddy's girl. He used to come down and see me every weekend when I was young (I lived with my granny) and I would cherish those weekends with him. He was so funny, and so manly, and so in control, and intelligent, and erudite; you can only be that funny when you're smart. I really looked up to him and admired him.

The first time I noticed something was a bit awry was when he called me and said, 'I've just taken the underland train.' What he was trying to say was 'underground'; I was waiting for him to correct himself, but he never did. He just used completely the wrong word, and I thought, *Oh, that's a bit funny.* But then he did it again in the same telephone conversation. He used the wrong word. He said to me, 'Well, call me when your work's less explosive.' What he was trying to say was, Call me when you're less busy, but he couldn't think of how to say it. So I called my mum, Gaby, and said, 'I think something's up with Dad.' We had a big chat about it, then we started watching for these

slip-ups of language that he was having and began to piece together that there was a problem.

But now I think back to it, when we were on *The Million Pound Drop* (there was a celebrity one for charity and we were on it together), I remember at the time thinking that Dad seemed so different on that and, interestingly, it is how I would describe how I felt when I first had the symptoms of the perimenopause. He just didn't seem himself. He seemed a bit nervous, he seemed a little bit out of sorts, he didn't seem confident. He was always so confident but he felt a little bit lost, and that was not my dad. And I've never, in fact, until writing this book, thought about the similarities between what he was like when he started with Alzheimer's and what I was like when I started the perimenopause. I was not myself. I was out of sorts.

So these were all the red flags that we spotted. This progressed and his Alzheimer's affected his speech, so he could only say very few words and couldn't form sentences. And this erudite man, who was incredibly verbose, still wanted to talk – you could see he wanted to talk – but he just couldn't find any words at all.

So when I called my doctor, I was terrified that these feelings seemed so similar to what I'd seen Dad go through on *The Million Pound Drop*. There was me trying to find these words with the blank page there, which I talked about earlier. My doctor did listen to me and she was really, really sweet. She made me feel way better about it all.

But perimenopause is not just forgetfulness, it could be mood swings, or the rage ... This rage is shameful if you're a woman. To have rage come out of nowhere is very frightening and unsettling – not just for the people around you, but for you, too.

I had heart palpitations: I was strapped up to a heart monitor for a week; I was really worried about it. I spent a lot of time with my fingers on my pulse, thinking there was something seriously wrong.

There are many other side-effects that people suffer from that I didn't experience so much, like itchy skin, anxiety, depression, aching limbs, bleeding gums – all sorts of mouth, teeth and gum issues. And we don't talk about lots of these symptoms, because at our age, if you get an ache or a pain you kind of think, 'Oh well, maybe it's just growing older. Maybe this is just what happens.' Or you might look up your symptoms and think, 'Oh, well

my mum had arthritis, maybe it's arthritis.' Obviously the worst thing to do is to Google or go online to search blindly. If I Google heart palpitations, not good! I'll be there for twenty minutes, going, 'I'm literally going to have a heart attack.'

So, I'm hoping that if you read this book and you are a woman of perimenopausal or menopausal age, whatever age that might be, you might piece together some of these things and feel a bit better about some of your symptoms. Separately, heart palpitations are worth getting checked out anyway, but I want you to SEE and READ this book so you can recognise what's happening to you right now. And if it's not happening to you right now, then be prepared for what's coming round the corner, before it hits you. That's the dream.

Knowledge is power. I'm going to keep saying this, and I want you to have all the information that you need, because when you know it, you can own it. We've got it covered.

MENOPAUSE SYMPTOMS
YOU KNOW ... AND THE ONES
NO ONE TELLS YOU ABOUT

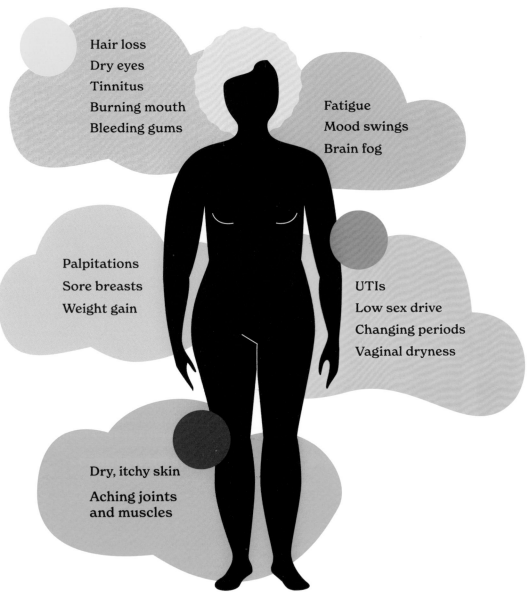

Hair loss
Dry eyes
Tinnitus
Burning mouth
Bleeding gums

Fatigue
Mood swings
Brain fog

Palpitations
Sore breasts
Weight gain

UTIs
Low sex drive
Changing periods
Vaginal dryness

Dry, itchy skin

Aching joints
and muscles

FEELING HOT HOT HOT (AND DEFINITELY NOT IN A GOOD WAY)

That feeling of FIRE. It's like some kind of comet travelling at a great pace throughout your body, which is burning hot. It can be just a sudden feeling, and I imagine a bit like a man with an erection – you never know when it's going to happen, there is no rhyme or reason to it, then suddenly you are on fire.

The most embarrassing things about it are: number one, the colour that it makes you go; and number two, that you just start sweating. Some people get the 'tache sweat, some people get the tit sweat – I mean, some people even get the crotch sweat. The crotch sweat is terrible. Why do we sweat in these places? This also stops women from wearing clothes that they want to wear for fear of sweat marks.

But I think the terrible, terrible thing about a hot flush is that when you're having one, it just isn't funny, and yet sometimes we kind of try to make an excuse about it and try to minimise it – 'Ooo I'm just having a hot flush!' – and people kind of joke about it. They think they're joking along with you but actually, it genuinely isn't funny, because when it's happening, all you can think about is what is happening in your body. You're not thinking about

the meeting, you're not thinking about the thing you've just said (you can't even remember the thing you just said because your face is on fire), you're not thinking about the date that you're on – you're not thinking about anything except just trying to get through this immensely uncomfortable moment.

I have to say that starting HRT was an absolute game-changer in terms of night sweats, and I would like to think that most women, if they're taking HRT, would be able to get their hot flushes completely under control.

There is a new medicine that is coming out that can really help with hot flushes. This too will be a game-changer for so many women, especially for those for whom HRT is not an option, because hot flushes really are debilitating.

'It was like someone had lit a fire in my belly.' — Nicola

An estimated eight out of ten women will get some kind of hot flush or night sweat[1], and lots of you have shared your stories of when and where these hot flushes strike, like Nicola, who had her first one at 40,000 feet.

I remember my first hot flush. It was four years ago when I was on a flight, I felt this burning rising from my stomach like someone had lit a fire in my belly. I told my husband to stand in the aisle and hide me while I took my trousers off.

OMG I was so embarrassed!

'It was horrible and embarrassing.' — Katie

Then there's Katie, who was told she was menopausal when she was just twenty-seven. Hot flushes were the first sign:

Where do I begin? I was twenty-six and I started waking up in the middle of the night soaking wet from sweating. It was horrible and embarrassing. I'd have to lie on a towel and change my pjs.

I thought it was because I'd recently moved house and it was better insulated than the last one, and therefore warmer.

I started getting random hot flushes during work at my desk and would look around to see if anyone else was hot, really confused. The gynaecologist broke the news to me when I was twenty-seven that I'd gone through the menopause.

It must have been such a horrible surprise to be told that at such a young age. Lots of love, Katie, and thanks for telling us your story.

---

[1] R. Bansal, N. Aggarwal (2019), 'Menopausal hot flashes: a concise review', *Journal of Mid-Life Health*, 10 (1), pp.6-13, doi.org/10.4103/jmh.JMH_7_19

AND NOW FOR THE SCIENCE BIT: WHY DO HOT FLUSHES HAPPEN?

It's thought that lack of oestrogen affects the hypothalamus, the part of the brain that helps regulate body temperature. When this is disrupted, the brain can think the body is overheating which causes blood vessels close to the surface of our skin to dilate to try to cool us down. This gives us the hot flush.

In addition, our bodies try to cool us down by making us sweat. Food and drink can also trigger hot flushes, or make them worse, such as alcohol, spicy food and even smoking.

COLD FLUSHES

Nope, believe me, you haven't left the freezer door open.

The opposite of a hot flush is very possible. A cold flush is a sudden onset of shivering, chills and an icy cold feeling through the body. A cold flush can immediately follow a hot flush, or can occur in isolation.

MENOPAUSE RAGE: IT'S SCARY, AND MOSTLY FOR THE WOMEN IT'S HAPPENING TO

I am really not a shouty person, and as I've said before, there were moments in my perimenopause when I really behaved in a way that upset me, and my kids. I think that for many of us – if we're usually quite passive and aren't shouty people and don't normally blow a gasket – it's very frightening when we suddenly Go.

These outbursts of rage for me, personally, often would just come out of nowhere and I'd go from nought to sixty; something that normally wouldn't bother me at all would just make me so angry. I would have to practise walking away and then coming back. It was scary.

It didn't happen all the time; it would come and go. But sometimes it would break out, often while I was trying to get the kids into the car on the school run, and I would feel so bad and I would look at their little faces because they'd be thinking, *Who is this?* I hated myself, and I didn't understand what was happening to me.

. . . .

'I feel like I've totally lost myself.' — Jac

One of the women who shared her story was Jac, who went into menopause because of treatment for breast cancer.

She describes being 'thrust into menopause' by chemo, and that for her the worst symptom by far was the mood swings.

I'd already had a few hot flushes prior to treatment, but after that finished, the symptoms came on hard and fast. Four years later I'm still struggling.

The worst symptom by far is the awful mood swings: feeling dead inside, and like I've totally lost myself.

I've complained a few times to my GP about the impact on my mood but they've tried to give me antidepressants, which I have declined because it's

menopausing that's killing my mood, and antidepressants are not what I want nor believe I need.

I can only liken the way I feel to as if my whole life pre-breast cancer was a drunken hoorah, and post-breast cancer/menopause I've now sobered up.

I feel like all of my happiness and joy has been sucked out. I have the odd day where I feel some pleasure, but all in all, I feel absolutely flat. I hate feeling like this and just want the old me back.

I feel doomed to be a grumpy, irritable old boot, and I'm only forty-nine :-(

This breaks my heart. I am so sorry that you feel like this, Jac. Big hug. If Jac's experience sounds familiar, many, many of you are going through this and you ARE NOT going crazy, I promise you.

We have lives that are so crazy and so busy, and look, there are plenty of reasons why we might seem stressed out.

But moods aren't always down to whatever job you do, or a tricky relationship, or trying to get the kids to school, or whatever you've got on your plate. Sometimes it is actually down to chemicals.

Oestrogen regulates brain neuro-transmitters. When this is disrupted it can impact on mood and wellbeing.

WHAT'S HAPPENING TO MY PERIODS?

My cycle was literally twenty-eight days, regular as clockwork. Then there were quite subtle changes, my periods would maybe last a day longer. So normally I'd be maybe three days, four days of bleeding, but then it became maybe four days and potentially a bit heavier. I was a bit unsure of what was happening as I'd always been so absolutely on the button, the same thing every month.

I didn't really know why that was happening, but obviously these changes are completely normal with perimenopause, because of all the hormone shifts.

If you suffer from PMS, do as Dr Naomi suggests and keep an eye on your usual symptoms – if things get worse, it could be an early sign of perimenopause.

It is entirely normal for periods to change during perimenopause and stop at the point of menopause. Periods can become more frequent or less frequent, and lighter as well as heavier. If yours do become heavier, or you experience bleeding between periods or after intercourse, please seek advice from your doctor.

DRY VAG AND OTHER SYMPTOMS TO DO WITH OUR VAGINAS

This is a BIGGY, but it is so rarely talked about and it is SO ABSOLUTELY VITAL for us to talk about because it is a really, really common symptom of perimenopause and the menopause. It is one that we do not talk about to each other because there is an embarrassment, there is an idea of, *oh is that what's causing it?*, or *there's probably nothing we can do about it*, or *maybe now that I can't have babies my vagina's just shut forever.* But it's NOT. And there's NO reason why we can't have lovely supple vulvas and vaginas for the rest of our lives. We just need to talk about the problem, because there is this really, really easy fix.

I didn't have the crippling issues that many women have with dry vaginas – UTIs, problems with incontinence and things like that – but I absolutely had a problem with dry vagina when it came to wiping myself after going to the loo. I just wasn't lubricated enough and I would wipe myself and it would start slightly catching, because there was no natural lubricant for the loo paper to swipe over. So I began to get really sore and every time I went to the loo it would sting. It was obviously the same for all areas of pleasure – self-pleasure and pleasure with my partner – that

would also become painful. HRT completely sorted that out for me but I am not ruling out the fact that if something does change and I do need a little bit of extra help, I can get that sorted very easily.

So oestrogen, basically, keeps the tissues of our vulva and vagina nice and supple. But oestrogen decline can cause these tissues to become thinner, lose their lubrication and become more painful. So, as I just said, the result – going to the loo, sex, sitting down – can really HURT. The lack of oestrogen is also very tricky with our waterworks, leading to problems like stress incontinence, which I definitely have had – so that when you laugh, or lift something heavy, wee comes out. Wanting to wee a lot at night-time was another issue, and this was the thing that mainly used to wake me up. So I would have broken sleep, for ages, which was unbelievably debilitating, because broken sleep means that you *never* get a proper night's sleep, which is not good for your brain function either. Low oestrogen levels can also make you a lot more prone to urinary tract infections – and you know how horrible those feel.

So look, if this sounds familiar to you, and you need some help and advice **right now**, skip this bit and go straight to Chapter 8: The Dry Vagina Monologues. It covers everything you need to know about how to spot, treat and beat vaginal dryness and UTIs.

Don't worry: it really IS all going to be ok.

SEX DRIVE M.I.A?

Oestrogen and testosterone are really important in terms of sexual function. During the perimenopause, when levels fluctuate, you may notice your libido take a nosedive. You might not be as sensitive to touch or just not feel in the mood as often, and this can particularly be the case if you have a surgical or medically-induced menopause (when your body goes into menopause because of medical treatment or surgery), because of the sharp decline in hormones.

And even if your mind's saying, *Yes, let's do it!* your body is saying *NO*. Vaginal dryness, as we talked about earlier, and symptoms like UTIs, can be a massive barrier to a happy sex life. And other things like hot flushes or that tyre that we put on around our waists overnight: all of these things are TERRIBLE for our self-esteem, which in turn is terrible for our libido.

Let's not forget how absolutely shattered we are, either, because we are up five times a night, weeing and sweating. And we have been on the go all day, with teenagers and kids, or a mad job – or all of it.

Often when you've got little kids, especially babies, your libido takes a hit. But when you go through perimenopause your libido can wane and you don't even really notice it – it happens quite slowly.

Before HRT, I felt that I'd changed so much physically, and I was SO tired from not sleeping. I was SO exhausted from waking up all those times during the night, that it really affected how I felt about my body, which in turn affected how I felt about sex.

Recently, I was talking to a mate going through the menopause. She's been with her husband for years and always had a super-healthy sex life; it had been a huge part of their relationship. She was so depressed because she felt that her libido had just disappeared, but her husband still had the same sex drive he'd always had, and he couldn't understand why she didn't want him anymore. He felt frustrated and rejected, unloved and confused. And she felt guilty, because she was shattered and didn't feel the same way as she used to and that was putting a huge strain on their relationship.

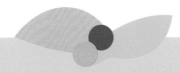

MENOPAUSE FROM A SOUTH ASIAN PERSPECTIVE, BY DR NIGHAT ARIF, NHS GP WITH A SPECIAL INTEREST IN WOMEN'S HEALTH

Contrary to what you may see in magazines and newspapers, menopause isn't a white, middle class, Western phenomenon.

In England and Wales, 14 per cent of the population are from ethnic minority backgrounds. Yet despite this, there is a lack of awareness, understanding and research on the experiences of menopause among minority communities.

As a GP, a British Muslim and as a woman, I'm keenly aware there is a whole host of reasons why menopause care for women in minority communities just isn't good enough.

First, menopause is a blind spot for many of my medical colleagues – many just haven't had the training to fully understand menopause and the impact it can have.

Secondly, if we look specifically at the experiences of ethnic minority women, there is the shame, stigma and taboo that surrounds women's health. In some communities, openly discussing periods or even just saying the word "vagina" out loud is virtually unthinkable.

Religion can also play a huge factor in seeking help. Some see health issues as a test from Allah or something you have to bear as a testament to your commitment to your faith.

Then there is the language barrier when seeking help. Women for whom English isn't their first language can struggle to express what their symptoms are. Menopause doesn't cross the language barrier in some cultures and women can find it hard to vocalise their symptoms in terminology Western-trained doctors will understand. In my native language Punjabi/Urdu there is no direct translation for the word 'menopause'. The closest word is *banjee*, which means 'barren'. Having to rely on relatives to translate just adds to the feelings of embarrassment.

Psychological symptoms of menopause such as low self-esteem or confidence do not always translate, while physical symptoms like aches and pains, dry eyes and tinnitus are things I hear about a lot from ethnic minority women. But because there is also a lack of awareness of menopause and understanding that it is linked to hormones, women may not make the link, and a Western-trained doctor could put pain down to something

like fibromyalgia and treat it as a musculoskeletal problem rather than menopause. In the West, a lot of the menopause rhetoric is around hot flushes but talking about hot flushes to a patient from Pakistan, where temperatures can reach 50°C, is very different.

So how can we change the conversation to make it more inclusive?

For me, Tik Tok has become an incredibly important tool to help educate people about menopause. I started doing videos during lockdown: with the focus on COVID-19, overnight all the women who would come and see me about menopause symptoms stopped coming and I wanted to find a way to reach them.

The beauty of Tik Tok is that it is short and shareable. I make bitesize videos that women themselves could watch, but also daughters and sons can show to their mothers, aunties, grandmothers and get the conversation going.

Sometimes I get shamed on social media from my own community, that what I am doing is somehow against Islam, or the topics I talk about should be kept private.

But change has to come from within, and if like me, you are Muslim or from a community where you aren't included in the mainstream menopause conversations, there are things you can do to empower not just yourself, but other women in your communities. We want our voices in the mainstream and not be seen as the 'other'.

Do your research and use it to help others. I'm a clinician using my skills to help people in Urdu and Punjabi, so if you have language skills, use them to educate those around you.

Normalise talking about menopause in your inner circles, to help stop those fatalist arguments like 'my mother had to bear it, so I should too' once and for all.

There should be no shame in talking about healthcare and nothing should be taboo.

Look at me: I'm a 38-year-old woman who loves Tik Tok. I've got absolutely no shame, because I'll be damned if our future daughters have to go through what our grandmothers, mothers and our peers and we ourselves have to go through.

And my final point. Embrace social media: don't be afraid of it! It can be a real force of good and a way to get the menopause message out there across the generations.

BRAIN FOG, AKA
'DID I SAY THAT ALREADY?'

It's always quite hard to explain to somebody who isn't going through perimenopause what brain fog means. We get to our mid-forties, or our early forties, or our late thirties, and we've lived quite a life. Sometimes we've got young children, sometimes we've got careers, sometimes we're organised members of society who help with charities. It doesn't really matter, but by the time you've got to that age, generally speaking you are quite *on it*. You are a valuable and productive member of society who is reliable, and when you are asked to do something, you turn up on time.

Brain fog, for me, was an absolute HORROR, because I am List Lady. I am super-organised. I am Madam Multi-tasker. And all of a sudden, I am literally just not turning up to a mate's supper somewhere. Like, not even remembering. I'd forgotten to put it in my diary, I'm not at my friend's supper, they all call me up and go, 'Where are you?' And they might have told me about it that morning, and I would have said to them, 'Yes, I'll see you tonight.' And I would have forgotten after putting the phone down. That is what brain fog is.

If you are a relative or a loved one of somebody who is suffering with brain fog, *it's not their fault.* It's the hormones. You might look at them and go, 'Really? You forgot that?' Or, 'Really? You didn't remember the thing I told you this morning?' Honestly: We. Don't. Remember.

The way I combat that stress is that I try to bring in immense order. Now that I've forgotten so many events, my diary is a very complex place where I just literally write down everything. I keep lots of notes in my phone to help me remember things that I think I might forget. I put in reminders a couple of days before somebody's birthday, even if it's normally a birthday that I would remember with ease every year.

I try to keep my life relatively in order. Things like: I get up, I make my bed, I tidy my house, because I feel like, 'tidy house tidy mind'. These little things do help me.

One morning, I was sitting on the drive and I looked at some grass, and I was thinking, what is the name of a big patch of green stuff like that? It's not grasses ... I could remember the word grass, and I was thinking, but when there's a lot of it together ... ? And I was thinking, *wow, there's nothing there.* The page was completely blank. I thought, *wow, this is really frightening, I don't even know what that is.* And about six hours later, I thought: *lawn! That's the word!*

Anybody who's reading this who has gone through that, don't worry – it happens to all of us, and there are lots of things that you can do to help yourself.

Brain fog is a kind of umbrella term for all those memory-related symptoms – forgetfulness, finding sentences, trailing off while you try to find the right word, or just feeling that your brain is stuck in first gear.

'I've got an English degree ... but I was struggling to find the right words.' — Joanne

A lot of you shared stories about how this has been a whopper issue for you at home, in relationships and at work, and Joanne very kindly got in touch and told us her story.

A single mum of two sons, she says she always prided herself on being 'fiercely independent and self-sufficient', but the brain fog left her struggling:

At forty-five I noticed that I was lacking energy and cognitively I didn't feel as sharp as normal. I've got a degree in English literature and language and yet I was struggling to find the right words.

As I'm very independent and have always felt confident in my academic and conversing abilities, this really unnerved me. I went from being linguistically confident to stumbling with words – it was scary.

I bet it was, Joanne. I bet it was really scary, because it was so out of character for you. And I think this is the frightening thing, when you think, *this isn't me. What has happened to me?*

So why does it happen? Well, oestrogen contributes to memory, cognition and verbal reasoning, so it's no wonder you might walk into a room and have no idea what you came in for. In fact, one study even shows menopause can affect tasks like remembering a short paragraph or a sequence of numbers.[2]

FATIGUE AND SLEEP DEPRIVATION: WHEN COUNTING SHEEP JUST WON'T CUT IT

The next symptom really, really floored me. It's awful. Lack of sleep is so detrimental to our wellbeing. It didn't just affect my mood, it affected my brain fog, it left me feeling frazzled, forgetful, annoyed, angry. You know, I need seven to eight hours of sleep a night, and I am famous for really annoyingly being able to put my head on a pillow, close my eyes and I'm literally out for the count straight away. But I was waking up six or seven times a night, often in the throes of a terrible night sweat and having to get up, change the sheets, then just about get back to sleep before waking up for a wee, feeling uncomfortable about

---

[2] Arun S. Karlamangla et al. (2017), 'Evidence for cognitive aging in midlife women: study of women's health across the nation, PLoS One, 12(1), doi.org/10.1371/journal.pone.0169008 PMCID: PMC5207430

the sheets and having to change them, as they would all be wet again.

Then the next morning, I'd look like some Shar-Pei puppy, and I wouldn't look even remotely normal until I'd literally slathered myself in moisturiser – so much that if you'd tried to hug me I'd slip out of your arms!

Hot flushes and night-time wees can shock even the heaviest sleeper out of a slumber, like me. Sleep problems can also be linked to anxiety, which can lead to waking up early or tossing and turning a lot, very light sleep, or waking several times a night. If I've had a couple of bad nights' sleep in a row, I am USELESS the next day. Do you know what I mean?

SPARE TYRE?

O.M.G. WHAT THE HELL happens during the menopause that means that virtually overnight you wake up and seem to have put on this little bit of meat around your middle? Why does that happen? Why is it the middle? What is going on?

It IS a thing. And the backfat, right? The backfat kind of by your bra strap? And what is happening to the little pockets of fat in your armpit, by your bra strap, going over your shoulder?

I mean, when I was young, I was one of those people who, if I ever put on weight and thought, *oh I can't get into my jeans*, I knew what I'd do. I literally would just work out a bit, or do three days of eating sensibly – and it was gone.

After I had children, I very publicly turned into the exercise lady. I met

Jackie and Mark and they revolutionised the way I looked and exercised, and I started exercising three times a week. And everything changed. Throughout my thirties I was the person who, when I did put on a bit of weight (I always did; I was quite a yo-yo person), I would just up the exercise and off it would fall.

I had massive babies – I mean, Chester was 10lb 2oz! – and while the tummy was massive, I did manage to work it off. But, oh my God, over the last few years I don't know what's happened but it is SO hard! I think it's metabolism – the way that we store fat changes, and we start to store more weight around our middles as we get older. Lovely child-bearing hips go, and hello spare tyre! This fat is really stubborn, too. It's as stubborn as a mule. And I know that many of us have struggled with weight gain at this time, and it is depressing. Often people say to me, 'Does HRT make you lose weight?' If I'm absolutely honest, it didn't for me, no. But what it DOES do is give you back the energy, and impetus, and the positive mindset that you need in order to exercise. It is complex, as it can allow weight loss if you find that your lifestyle factors change too (and this can even be without adding exercise).

I know it's hard, and it just kind of adds to that sense of feeling invisible when we hit menopause. But it's also really bad for our long-term health if we let that spread. Carrying weight around our middle puts us at an increased risk of diabetes, heart disease and cancer.

So later we're going to talk about exercise, and how we can try to find the energy and the enthusiasm to exercise again to keep that weight off the middle. I'm not talking about running marathons, I'm talking about stuff that all of us can do – and maintain.

ELBOWS, SHOULDERS, KNEES AND TOES

'Elbows, shoulders, knees and toes, knees and toes…' I know that's not quite how the song goes, but it is the best way I can describe what I'm next going to talk about, which is all those little niggly aches and pains that suddenly seem to start happening once we hit perimenopause.

As I mentioned before, I had my babies, and I started exercising, and I got really uber-fit. I was known for my fitness and I really enjoyed exercising. Then all of a sudden I'd get a little pull somewhere, a little tweak in my calf muscle. I pulled the tendons in the tops of my fingers on each hand a couple of times, and that was a twelve-week recovery.

We are going to get twinges, and we are going to feel creaky, and we might make hurrrh noises when we bend down to put our shoes on, BUT bear in mind that all of these things aren't necessarily **just** getting older. It could be menopause.

Oestrogen is a bit like WD40 for our joints and muscles. It keeps them supple and flexible.

About half of women will experience joint pain around menopause.[3]

'I know my own body, and something wasn't right.' — Lorraine

For Lorraine – a personal trainer who shared her story – aches and pains were the first sign that something had changed:

I knew something was going wrong with my body when I started getting pains in my Achilles, knees and shoulders. As a PT and endurance enthusiast, I know my own body, and something wasn't right.

Then the anger and anxiety arrived, like a dark cloud over my usual positive self. Luckily, I did my research and pushed my GP, and after two years of being offered antidepressants, MRI scans and cortisone injections, I was finally given HRT. Had I not done my research I would never have known what was happening.

I will ALWAYS speak out and help to educate and support others who may not have the same fight as me … we should not suffer this awful thing alone. x

Lorraine, thank you so much for saying you will always speak out and educate. You are amazing and we absolutely should support each other and not suffer alone. You are totally right.

THUMPING HEADACHES

Now, I have been very lucky because I've never really suffered with this, but I know lots and lots of women that do. If all these symptoms are giving you a bit of a headache, you might be onto something, because fluctuating hormones can be linked to more frequent and more painful migraines, and perimenopause and menopause are no exception.

---

[3] M. Magliano (2010). 'Menopausal arthralgia: Fact or fiction', Maturitas, 67(1) pp. 29-33, doi.org/10.1016/j.maturitas.2010.04.009

If you've suffered from migraines previously, they might become more frequent and more intense. Or you might find that you are experiencing them for the first time. If you've suffered migraines during hormone fluctuations in the past, such as during puberty, when you were taking the contraceptive pill, or during pregnancy, you might find you're more susceptible. HRT when used in the correct regime generally does not make migraines worse and can improve them.

'I thought I had a brain tumour.' — Victoria

When Victoria started having irregular periods at the age of thirty-nine, she thought she might be pregnant. But then the night sweats started, along with a headache that just wouldn't shift.

The headaches were usually more painful down one side, so much so that I thought I was developing a brain tumour. Words started to escape me in the middle of sentences, so I made a conscious effort not to start a conversation in the first place for fear of looking stupid.

I went to my GP and asked if my hormone levels were ok. The GP thought I could be too young to be perimenopausal. I also went about my headaches but it was still not investigated as a symptom of perimenopause. I started to think that I was perimenopausal, just by simply talking to other people and reading up on it. I couldn't compare to my own

mother because she had no symptoms, and I felt quite alone with it at times. I also had high levels of anxiety, not trusting my own judgement and writing everything down because I'd forget easily. I very nearly asked about antidepressants because I felt like I didn't know what to do with myself.

But in the end, I knew I didn't need them. I finally plucked up the courage to go back to the GP five years after symptoms first began – and I'm now on HRT. Fingers crossed I will be able to feel the full benefits of it soon – I've only been on it twelve days as I type this.

Victoria talks about having irregular periods when she was thirty-nine, which is very, very early but not impossible, and more and more women I talk to show signs of perimenopause before they're forty. Do not ignore these signs.

Thank you for sharing your story, Victoria, and I really hope you start feeling the benefits of HRT, because to basically lose five years due to your symptoms – that's tough. I do hope the oestrogen panned out. If you have been put on HRT and you're not feeling the benefits at all, doctors often start you on very low dosages, so it's always worth going back to talk to your GP about the dosage that you're on, and to ask if you can go on a higher dosage if you're not feeling any benefits.

LET'S TALK BOOBS

When I was pregnant, my boobs grew massively. I mean, I would go from a B to a D overnight like they'd been inflated with a balloon pump. And the same thing started happening at the start of perimenopause. I had no idea what it was about, but actually of course it's down to hormones again.

There's something about hormone-inflated boobs that makes me feel really old. They're not all swollen to provide milk, which is a useful thing for your baby. When I got really big, swollen, achy, menopausal boobs, it just made me feel **old**. I can't really explain why; I'm sure some of you will relate. But because my hormones were all over the place, I had fluid retention which made them go up and down, and up and down, and at times during my perimenopause my boobs would hurt like hell. And let's just discuss the bra sizes! My boobs would grow one or two sizes – who can have three different sizes of bra in their drawers? That gets expensive.

What happens is that when you get near menopause your oestrogen levels plummet, your breasts start to change from milk-makers to the next phase. Don't be depressed about this. Your boobs can be just as much fun after they've stopped being milk-makers.

The tissue in your breast starts to shrink, and becomes less elastic, and you might notice that your boobs have become less pert, and saggier. I mean, they'd started becoming less pert and saggier the minute I'd had babies, but this is also a sign of menopause, and perimenopause. While we're on the subject, if you don't already, please, by the way, check your boobs regularly. You can never check your boobs enough. Every day. Every time you're in the shower – just do it.

I'm obsessed with my bathroom. It's a place of peace and quiet for me. The way that I relax and chill out is I have a long soak in the bath to unwind, with tons of Badedas bubble bath. (I'm a child of the seventies and it really reminds me of my childhood. I don't know what they put in that stuff; it's literally lime green, but the smell of it just reminds me so much of, I don't know ... happy days.) I like a bath in the evening, and sometimes, if I'm going to work, I'll have a shower in the morning. But I'm checking my boobs all over the place – shower, bath, wherever. Wherever there's water, I'm checking my boobs.

See nbcf.org.au, or the UK's NHS website has a really good guide to checking your breasts.[4]

KNOW what's normal for your boobs.

LOOK at your breasts and FEEL them.

KNOW what changes to look for – this can include puckering or dimpling, a rash or redness.

REPORT any changes to your GP without delay.

GO to routine screening if you're aged fifty to seventy.

---

[4] NHS.uk (2021), 'How should I check my breasts?', www.nhs.uk/common-health-questions/womens-health/how-should-i-check-my-breasts/

ELECTRIC SHOCK SENSATION

This isn't a symptom that I've ever had, but I've spoken to friends of mine and they say it is a really weird sensation and not one that they had ever associated with perimenopause or menopause. It's a bit like getting elastic bands twanging under your skin, and it can also be associated with restless leg syndrome, or you can feel like they are twanging under your hair, in your arms, in your legs. It can happen on its own, it can be a bit of a precursor to a hot flush, but it's very annoying. It often happens in bed, and it's about the messages that go between your nervous system and your brain. And sometimes they misfire.

PALPITATIONS

I talked about this earlier, and this is a feeling that's really frightened me, because my heart would feel like it was *pounding* so fast, and sometimes it would kind of skip a beat, like it would have an arrhythmia or something.

Palpitations can happen for all sorts of reasons – excitement, stress, caffeine, smoking – but these, when I had them, would happen to me when I was sat down without a coffee or a tea, just watching television. I ended up going to see a doctor about it and wearing a heart monitor for a few days. But what I didn't know – and this was at a time when I knew about most symptoms for the perimenopause, and I'd been on HRT for a while – is that changing hormone levels can increase your heart rate and palpitations can coincide with this. And sometimes with hot flushes.

Obviously, if you're having palpitations, be cautious. Get it checked out. Talk to your doctor. Mine definitely were connected to the menopause because I had everything checked; I got thoroughly looked over. It wasn't anything serious to worry about and, interestingly, they've gone away now, so it would make complete sense that they were hormonal.

If you are worried, go see your doctor.

BLEEDING GUMS OR BURNING MOUTH?

Problems with your mouth, teeth and gums are much more common than you think. Declining oestrogen levels can result in a drop in saliva production, which can cause women a parched, dry mouth, and what some women sometimes describe as a 'burning mouth'. Women have told me they can sometimes feel like their whole tongue or mouth is on fire.

But sometimes it's more subtle than that. It can be just that feeling of less saliva, that leaves you feeling like you just want to swoosh a bit of water around in your mouth, or tea, or get a drink or whatever in you.

But what happens is that when you've got less saliva in your mouth, it literally is like a breeding ground for nasties to come and hang out. Bacteria that would normally get swished around and removed sit for longer on the gums, and it can lead to bad breath, and even tooth loss.

Now, lots of women suffer with dental problems and oral issues with the menopause, and they don't know that this is a symptom – but it is. Stress, tiredness, anxiety and depression can make it worse.

. . . .

'My burning tongue and mouth ulcers affected my everyday life.' — Jan

Here's Jan – she's shared her story with us. She had anything up to forty mouth ulcers at any time, and she lost her sense of taste and smell.

I haven't had the usual symptom of hot flushes like my friends, instead I suffered

with a burning tongue and mouth ulcers. As my GP said I was not menopausal, I wasn't able to access HRT or other treatments/replacements.

I am now post-menopausal: I no longer have a burning tongue, but I still suffer with mouth ulcers and loss of taste and smell. I find it difficult as no one offered me support or help.

When I discuss it with my friends, they say I am 'lucky'. But the symptoms I had were very painful and affected my daily life. Menopause affects women in different ways and I want other women to know that it can be stressful even if you do not display the 'usual' symptoms.

Thank you for talking about this, Jan; it is really important to talk about these different symptoms, because you are not alone. Many women will be going through this and might not have any other type of symptom, but this is absolutely a symptom of menopause, and HRT can help with it – it's not just to lubricate your vagina, but your mouth as well.

THE (DRY) EYES HAVE IT

What's really interesting is that I went to the optician the other day, to have my eyes tested, and she said to me, 'Oh, you've got dry eyes.' I've never had that before, but this is a symptom that I'd developed over the last few years. My eyes didn't feel gritty, or sore, but she did say that it is important to keep your eyes lubricated.

Every time we blink we leave a thin layer, called a tear film, which helps keep our eyes nice and moist and comfortable, and our vision clear. Dry-eye syndrome **can** make you feel gritty and sore, but it can be something that you're not aware that you have. That's why it is really useful to still go and see an optician, especially when you're perimenopausal or menopausal. Dry-eye syndrome is

when they feel tired, or itchy, or – weirdly – sometimes they can water a lot – especially in cold or windy weather, so you look like you're crying, which is what I had.

The risk of having dry eyes increases with age, but perimenopause and menopause put us at further risk, because oestrogen plays a part in the production of the tear film. So when oestrogen declines, our eyes can feel dry.

There are things you can do: you can make sure that your lids, and inside your lids, stay nice and clean, and there are eye drops you can get for it that will help you with that, so it is treatable.

DRY, SORE AND ITCHY SKIN

Oh good God. I had this SO bad.

You know what, collagen's an amazing thing – it's like a building block for our bodies. It strengthens our bones and our muscles and our skin, and our hair, and it gives them structure. And do you know what is crucial in collagen production? Go on, guess… YES! You're right. OESTROGEN. It's crazy how important oestrogen is.

Look, I'm not all pert like I was when I was twenty. I've got laughter lines, crow's feet, my face is thinner. If you've noticed that your skin is looking a bit saggy and more wrinkled, and less smooth – don't give yourself a hard time. Your skin's just feeling the effects of diminishing collagen.

Studies show that skin loses about a third of its collagen during the first five years of menopause.[5] And it's not just collagen that we wave goodbye to, we're also losing the fatty lipid layer that sits on the skin barrier and protects. And because that layer is compromised, we lose more water via the skin, which can leave the skin dry, dull, flaky and more sensitive.

If your skin is suffering, fear not – the AMAZING skincare guru Caroline Hirons has some foolproof, no-nonsense skincare tips a little later on in the book (see page 274).

… AND WHAT ABOUT SPOTS?

As if wrinkly, sagging skin and jowls wasn't bad enough, you might also have spots to contend with (wah!). With oestrogen on the wane, androgens – a collective term for male hormones like testosterone – start to take centre stage. Androgens stimulate glands in our skin called sebaceous glands, making them produce more oil or sebum. Our pores become blocked, et voilà – say hello to spotty, oily skin.

---

[5] American Academy of Dermatology Association (2021), 'Caring for your skin in menopause', www.aad.org/public/everyday-care/skin-care-secrets/anti-aging/skin-care-during-menopause

ENOUGH TO MAKE YOUR SKIN CRAWL

It may sound like something you get up to in the bedroom, but formication is the name for a sensation of ants crawling on your skin. The scalp and calves are most often affected, and again it all comes back to oestrogen and the depletion of the fatty lipid layer on the skin.

'Everything itched or ached.' — Angeline

Angeline shared her story about being just thirty-five when her periods stopped. She struggled with hourly hot flushes that would strike any time, and itchy skin.

I wanted to rip my skin off. How could I burn this much on the inside every thirty or forty minutes, day and night? It was relentless.

Everything itched or ached. My libido died. My marriage struggled. Insomnia started and I managed on three–five hours of broken sleep a night.

Angeline, thank you for sharing your story. It's absolutely horrific, isn't it, the way that one thing in your body – one change in your body – can ruin your life. And I hope you have found a way to help yourself through that. If you haven't, keep reading, because we might be able to help you later on in the book.

MORE THAN JUST A BAD HAIR DAY

Brittle hair that breaks when you run a brush or your fingers through it? Hair just doesn't seem to grow, or that is even falling out?

Declining oestrogen can affect the texture of our hair, leading to breakage and a receding hairline, especially around the temples. On the flip side, you might find you are sprouting more facial hair – it's those androgens (male hormones like testosterone) taking centre stage again.

If you notice specific hair loss patterns or areas of baldness, you should go and see your doctor.

RINGING EARS

Tinnitus is the term for any ringing, buzzing or whooshing sounds in one or both of your ears. At best it is an inconvenience that comes and goes, at worst it can be debilitating and disrupt your everyday life. About one in eight people in the UK suffers from tinnitus and, guess what, it can be more common in perimenopause and menopause. Sadly, the exact cause isn't yet known.

I got Covid and had tinnitus as a result of that, and since then I have occasionally had a little bit of ringing in my ears, and it's very frustrating. I don't know whether mine was because of perimenopause or because of Covid, but if you suffer from tinnitus, I'm relating and sympathising in a big way. If you have any concerns, always go and see your doctor.

HISTAMINE INTOLERANCE

Until I met Dr Naomi I'd never even *heard* of this symptom, but I reckon it's something we are going to be hearing more and more about over the next few years. A growing area of research is the interaction between oestrogen and histamine levels. Histamine is a chemical we produce when the body thinks it's under threat from foreign invaders, but it is also found in foods like tomatoes, avocados, pulses, dairy, alcohol and caffeine.

But what does this have to do with perimenopause and menopause, I hear you say? It's thought that fluctuating hormone levels may interfere with the way we get rid of the histamine, or lead to overproduction of histamine. There are loads of symptoms linked to histamine intolerance and a lot of them crossover with other perimenopause and menopause symptoms, such as hives, itchy skin, headaches, joint pain, fatigue and urinary symptoms like cystitis (inflammation of the bladder that triggers that awful burning sensation when you have a wee). Histamine intolerance can also trigger shortness of breath, a sore throat, stuffy nose and cough.

The issue of histamine sensitivity is a recently identified phenomenon and only just becoming widely known. The paradox is that in perimenopause, lower levels of oestrogen seem to trigger histamine sensitivity, but treating lower oestrogen levels can also trigger histamine intolerance. Women with these symptoms find accessing the appropriate care challenging but treatment generally involves cautious use of HRT and the lowering of histamine triggers, including possible dietary changes.

WAYS TO BECOME MORE VISIBLE

The problem is, as we hit perimenopause and menopause, we feel like we literally disappear overnight. That we become irrelevant, invisible, uninteresting, unattractive to society. Now, I think that the French seem to have it right, because I feel like French women are totally badass. Even in their seventies, I see women strutting about like they are literally the dog's bollocks. And it's not that they have got pert skin, or that they have had loads of plastic surgery and look really young, or that they are dressing in a way that is showing off: it's that they are oozing confidence.

When you ooze that kind of confidence, people just see you, but the problem is, when you hit perimenopause and menopause, it's like somebody has just literally emptied out your confidence reserve. They've just taken it, and they've thrown it away. And you are left with nothing. So I've got some tips on how to build your self-confidence, how to feel better about yourself. These are small things, but I promise you they are going to help.

The first thing is: **start with your underwear**. Ladies, I am telling you, it is not ok to wear the grey underwear that was white five years ago, that's sightly frayed around the edges, that's not matching. You've got non-matching bras and pants and it's all very comfortable looking, and you put it on because you think, well, nobody's going to see it, what's the point? Uh ... *hello?* YOU see it. This is not ok! You are worth wearing matching underwear, or nice underwear, or underwear that's clean. I'm not talking about underwear that's going to cost you a fortune. Listen, there are some amazing companies out there making really pretty underwear that does not cost the earth. Twice a year, don't just buy yourself a new pair of jeans. You wear underwear every single day; it's the one staple. You will wear a bra and pants every. Single. Day.

So I've got some tips for you. When you buy your bra, buy three pairs of matching pants. It means that you will be able to wear matching underwear for three days (because you wear your bra three times, and you want clean pants to go with your bra). And, NEVER, EVER wash your white underwear with anything that's not white! Never let it go grey. I'm afraid, ladies, if it goes grey, you chuck it out. Get rid of the idea that underwear is for a man, or for a partner, or for your girlfriend – that's NOT ok. You should be wearing nice underwear for YOU, because YOU are worth it. I have my I-mean-business underwear. I have I-feel-frisky underwear – and that isn't for a man, that's for ME. I will get up in the morning and I'll think, *oo I feel frisky today*, and I will put on my I-feel-frisky underwear. It's about YOU and pleasing YOU.

So feeling visible starts with **you** feeling that **you** want to see **yourself**. I want you to put your underwear on and I want you to look in the mirror in the morning, and I want you to think to yourself, 'Actually, I look rather nice.' That is how you are going to start your day.

Then I suggest that every day you wear something that is a little bit out of character for you. So, are you the type of person who only ever wears navy blue, white, grey and black? If you are, then wear a red shirt. Wear a red silk shirt that fits your form, that is a little bit va-va-voom. Or buy a pair of reading glasses that are **not** black or grey, that are perhaps leopard print. I'll tell you what, Karen Arthur has an Instagram account @menopausewhilstblack, and there's another Instagram @luinluland, which may help you to step out of your comfort zone in terms of what you are wearing. Luinluland takes that to another level. Or buy a pair of sunglasses that are screaming LOOK AT ME! Buy sunglasses that make you look like a rock star.

Do not give in to your brain telling you to be invisible because that's how you feel about yourself. Because when you put on those glasses, or the red shirt, or the crazy boot with a dress combo that you would never normally do, you're not doing it for anybody else, you're doing it for the way it makes YOU feel, and the way that it makes you smile to yourself. That inner, wry smile where you think, *oo get me, what am I doing?* Now, it might take you a while to build up to the kind of confidence that Karen or Lu have, but you'll get there. It doesn't mean that you will always have to wear stuff that's completely outrageous, but you will start really enjoying – as Karen says – wearing your happy. When you step out of your norm, people will go, 'Oh wow, I love your glasses,' or, 'Wow, I love that jumper!'

Try to never say, 'Oo, I could never wear that.' Or, 'I'm too old to wear that.' You are **never** too old to wear something! Be adventurous. It's exciting, and it will really put you in a good mood.

The next thing is: **walk with purpose**. When you feel invisible, the temptation is to walk invisibly. But what I want you to do is think about your posture, think about your shoulders, think about your head position. Keep your head up, look straight forward, and pick up the pace to wherever you're going.

Firstly because, actually, exercise is really good for you. Picking up the pace and not shuffling along is a positive thing that's good for your bones, it's good for your heart, it's good for everything. But also because it's like saying, 'Look at me.' I think we're embarrassed to say 'Look at me', but don't be! You're gorgeous. I want to see you. Shoulders back, head up, in your new pair of glasses, in your new shoes, or wearing something that you saw in a fashion magazine that you thought you'd be too old to wear, but you've done it anyway ... Be confident about it: hold your shoulders back, hold your head up high, and **walk with purpose**.

Another thing is: **stay relevant**. There is a temptation as we get older to feel like there is a certain type of music that belongs to young people. My passion is music, but I still listen to Radio 1 because I love to know what's coming out, what's new. I'm very lucky as my kids love music, too. They educate me all the time, they are always sending me tracks that they think I'd like. I love hearing about new DJs, I love hearing about new types of music that I might not know about.

I want to stay relevant. Not so I can try to be young, but so that if a kid talks to me about something, I can feel like, yeah, I know what you're talking about. But if the kids talk to me about a track, a singer that I haven't heard of, I love it when they tell me about it. And I try to remember it in case somebody else talks about it, or maybe play it to someone and introduce other people to a great new artist. I love all of that. Podcasts are also brilliant. I might want to learn about more celebrities, current affairs, expert interviews or business; it's a great way of educating myself. Staying relevant is just about keeping up to date, and never saying to myself, 'Oh I've got no idea about that, I'm too old to know about that.'

Age is a number. We can ALL learn new things, and sometimes I surprise myself. I learn about something new and might develop a real interest in or passion for something that I hadn't even known about before. Right now I'm obsessing about the metaverse; it's really blowing my mind, I'm fascinated with it and I'm learning something new about it every day. Never stop learning.

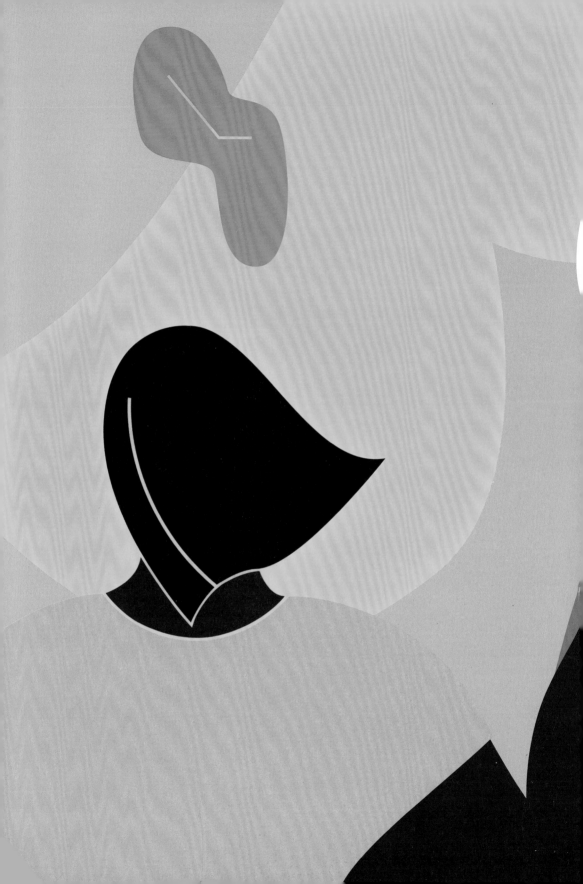

CHAPTER 4

EARLY MENOPAUSE AND PREMATURE OVARIAN INSUFFICIENCY

Early menopause.
It's MORE COMMON
than you might think.

1 in every 100 women go into menopause before they are 40.

1 in every 1,000 go into menopause before they are 30.

1 in every 20,000 go into menopause before they are 20.[1]

All too often we look at menopause through a midlife lens – look at me, I thought I was too young to be perimenopausal at the age of forty-four.

I now know that's only half the story. For tens of thousands of women, menopause happens much earlier than the average age of fifty-one. And when it happens years or even decades earlier than you expect, it can feel like a particularly cruel double whammy. Life is just getting exciting – finding your feet in your career, having fun with friends, new relationships ... and then you find out you're menopausal.

. . . .

'It's a relief to get a diagnosis.' — Sue

This chapter is for Sue and the thousands of other women out there going through early menopause. Sue is thirty-three, and when she shared her story, she'd just had it confirmed she was in early menopause:

It started for me August 2020, with tropical moments in the evening, hair loss, constant greasy hair, broken sleep, mood swings and memory loss. I only decided to speak with a doctor once my periods started to change: late, early, shorter, longer. I'd been on the pill for a number of years so I knew that shouldn't be happening.

I spoke to a lovely doctor. I told them 'I feel like I am going mad and losing my mind, help me!' And the response I got was, 'You're not going mad, we will help you.'

It's taken seven months to be diagnosed, after scans and blood tests. But I can honestly say it's a relief to be diagnosed and to know I'm not nuts.

Thank you, Sue, for sharing your story with us. Early menopause is a very lonely place to be, because you have so few people to talk to. But don't worry, we are all here for you.

[1] The Daisy Network (2021), 'What is POI?', www.daisynetwork.org/about-poi/what-is-poi

'I didn't tell anyone as I was ashamed.' — Natasha

Like Sue, so many of you have reached out with your stories of what it is like to go through an early menopause, including Natasha, who went into menopause at the age of just thirteen.

Natasha says she was too ashamed to tell anyone that she'd never had a period. It wasn't until she met her now-husband at the age of twenty-five that she reached out for help.

I didn't tell anyone as I was ashamed and thought I was a weirdo. I also developed erosive lichen planus [a rare skin disease that causes painful ulcers in the genitals], had a total hysterectomy and a vaginectomy.

I think I have had every menopause symptom known to mankind, I'm still struggling and having yearly surgery to divide the fused labia skin.

I'm now forty-five and I've only just been prescribed testosterone. It's been a hell of a journey. I'm on HRT (patches and gel) and vitamin D supplements as I have osteoporosis.

Premature ovarian insufficiency (POI) has to be talked about. It is a must in this day and age, so that no more young girls suffer in silence the way I did.

Natasha, literally my heart aches for everything that you have been through. I cannot imagine the trauma. I have spoken to women online about erosive lichen planus, and it is phenomenally painful, debilitating and difficult. So thank you so much for sharing that with us; you have helped so many women.

The idea that you've had to deal with early menopause at thirteen and then not been able to really talk to anybody about it until you met your partner when you were twenty-five – I hate the idea of any woman feeling alone, or such an extraordinary case that she doesn't feel like there's anybody else there in the world who could be going through the same thing as her. I really hope that reading some of the examples in this book will help, and that anyone – whether women, trans men or non-binary – can identify with something in here, and that everybody is represented.

A lot of you who got in touch spoke so passionately about the need for early menopause to be talked about more, so in this chapter, we'll be covering:

→ Why early menopause is more common than you think.

→ How to spot it, what to do about it – and why treatment is SO incredibly important for your future health.

→ Your early menopause stories: how you were diagnosed and how you got through it.

To all of you out there:

You are visible.

. . . .

You are important.

. . . .

You are heard.

WHAT IS AN EARLY MENOPAUSE AND WHY DOES IT HAPPEN?

So, we know the average age of menopause is fifty-one. 'Early menopause' describes menopause under the age of forty-five. Menopause under the age of forty is known as premature ovarian insufficiency (POI). As the stats at the start of this chapter show, early menopause and POI are more common than you think – one in 100 women will go through POI menopause before the age of forty.

So why does it happen? It's not always known exactly what causes POI, but in most cases it is down to one of the reasons described below:

In most cases we don't actually know why women go into early menopause, but these are some of the possible reasons.

Autoimmune conditions, where your immune system mistakenly thinks a part of your body is a foreign invader and starts to attack rather than protect it. There are any number of autoimmune conditions that affect many organ systems including thyroid, skin, hair and joints. There is a correlation with women who have POI and other autoimmune conditions.

Genetic conditions, one of the most common of which is Turner syndrome. Genetic conditions like Turner syndrome are more likely to be the cause of POI if you are very young at diagnosis.

Cancer treatment, such as chemo or radiotherapy to your pelvic area which causes temporary or permanent damage to the ovaries.

Surgery where the ovaries are removed, which could be due to a number of reasons, for example a painful condition where tissue similar to the lining of the uterus begins growing in places such as the ovaries. Surgical menopause tends to give more extreme symptoms as the source of the hormones is removed overnight.

Infections causing early menopause are rare, but there have been cases where mumps, malaria, HIV or tuberculosis have been identified as the cause.

I was actually diagnosed with hypothyroidism about twenty years ago. I went to my doctor to have my bloods checked, because I knew I was going to start trying for a baby; they flagged up that I had hypothyroidism and said that potentially if I didn't get it looked at, it might affect my ability to get pregnant. So they put me on a dose of levothyroxine, and I'd take that every day, and I have done for the last twenty years.

When I got pregnant, they upped the dosage, because you need a little bit more then, but normally I take 100 micrograms of levothyroxine every day, and that just replaces the thyroxine.

This has actually worked really well for me. I started going through perimenopause. I noticed it properly with the sweats at forty-four – but I do think possibly that things had started to go a bit awry with my hormones a couple of years before that, at forty-two. So that is a little bit early in terms of the age medical professionals would normally expect me to go through the menopause.

Interestingly, hypothyroidism is something that does need to get taken into account when looking at whether a woman is perimenopausal or not.

. . . . . .

'My friends were talking contraception and sex ... I was embarking on a journey nobody really understood.' — Aoife

Aoife was twenty-one when she was diagnosed with POI – or POF (premature ovarian failure), as it was called at the time. In her story, she talked about how that word – failure – haunted her for years.

There was no clear reason why she had POI, but her consultant thought it was probably because of an autoimmune disease.

She says she realised the significance of the diagnosis when her consultant told her it would be unlikely she would be able to conceive naturally. Later, when Aoife was in a relationship, there were conversations about egg donation, but she says she didn't feel ready to consider this. She started taking HRT when she was twenty-four.

I don't think I was at an age where I really understood how much this would impact my life. I loved children and wanted at least four! When I think back to when my symptoms started, I can remember being in secondary school and suffering with hot flushes. Life was tough, especially as not many doctors in Ireland, where I'm from, had come across anybody as young as I was who was going through this ... no one could help me, and my symptoms gradually became worse.

I felt so lonely. At a time when my friends were talking contraception and sex, I was embarking on a journey that I felt nobody really understood. However, I gave it a go and began to slowly feel better. Miraculously, when I was twenty-six, I fell pregnant. I was over the moon and cherished every day of my pregnancy, knowing how precious it was. I came off HRT straight away and carried my daughter to full term.

I tried to avoid going back on HRT, in the hope that I was no longer menopausal. But when symptoms like extreme tiredness, anxiety and aches in my joints returned with a bang, I started to take it again.

So, I have been on HRT now for thirteen years. It is life-changing and, when the dose and type of HRT that you are prescribed is correct, it is possible to feel like 'yourself' again. Patches saved me! I love to exercise and to live life to its fullest and I need HRT for that.

Menopause can be an incredibly lonely time for many women, and a premature menopause, even more so. Find a doctor that understands. For those of you that may be suffering, know that you are not alone and that there is so much support out there for you.

Aoife, thank you so much for telling us your story, and thank you for your inspirational end to your story. It is an incredibly difficult time for so many women, and premature menopause, you're right, is even more so, because so few women go through that. There is a lot of support out there – just go online and find other people in the same situation. We have listed some Instagram accounts and pages to follow if you do have POI (see page 300).

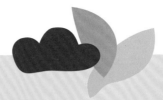

DR NAOMI:
GETTING A DIAGNOSIS OF
EARLY MENOPAUSE OR POI

Hearing a diagnosis of POI or early menopause can be unexpected and upsetting. In addition it can have health repercussions if not treated, so it is important that diagnosis is not delayed.

If you are between forty and forty-five years old, your doctor should be discussing your symptoms, medical history and family history (early menopause can sometimes, but not always, run in families) and look to rule out any other potential causes for your symptoms. You should be offered a blood test to check your FSH and oestradiol levels. Your doctor will likely do other investigations to exclude other causes of your symptoms such as thyroid function tests, vitamin D, full blood count and so on.

Hormone blood tests are snapshots of your hormone levels on any given day, so the test should be repeated about six weeks later to get a better picture. Please remember that even blood tests that come back 'normal' don't necessarily rule out a diagnosis and treatment can still be appropriate if you have typical symptoms but normal bloods.

If you are under forty, you will need more extensive investigations, so ideally your doctor should be referring you to a menopause clinic where they are experienced in caring for women with POI. You may also have other tests. These are to rule out other causes for symptoms and to look for a cause of POI. They will usually include tests such as autoimmune screening, thyroid function test, hormone profile and genetic testing. You may have a pelvic ultrasound scan to look at your ovaries, uterus and vagina. You should also be offered a bone density scan, known as a DEXA scan. This scan looks for signs of bone thinning and osteoporosis, because an early menopause can increase the risk of osteoporosis.

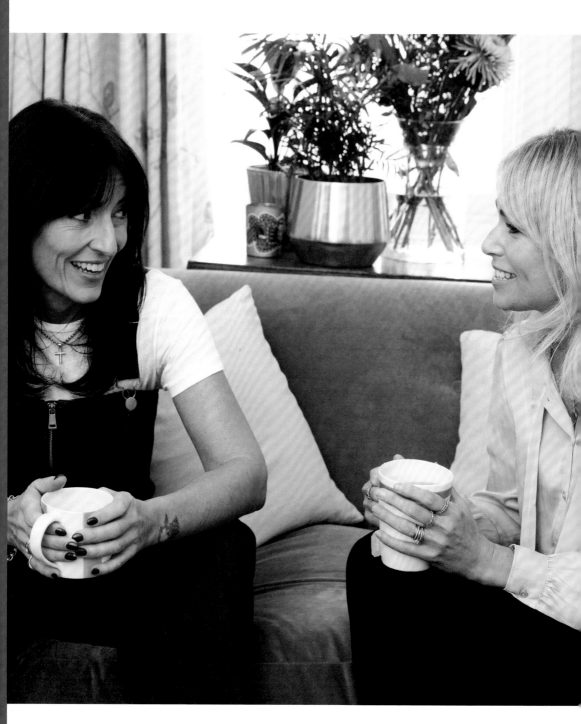

WHAT CAN BE THE SIGNS OF POI?

You might experience any menopausal symptoms, but these are the ones which may help you identify POI if you are under forty:

→ Missed or irregular periods

→ Problems getting pregnant

→ Low libido

→ Hot flushes and/or night sweats

→ Mood swings/worsening PMS

→ Vaginal dryness or soreness

→ Recurring urinary tract infections

WHY EARLY TREATMENT IS SO KEY

POI can occur at any age, even as young as the early teens. Because there is so little awareness of the condition, it can go undiagnosed for years but it's so important it is identified early to protect overall health.

As we will be covering in the next couple of chapters, HRT is the first-line treatment for menopause. It helps with symptoms, but also has an important, long-term protective effect against health problems like osteoporosis and cardiovascular disease.

Getting a diagnosis of early menopause, particularly POI, is so important because having depleted oestrogen levels at an earlier age puts you at greater risk of long-term problems like osteoporosis and cardiovascular disease.

The current guidance for healthcare professionals from the National Institute of Health and Care Excellence (NICE) is that women with POI or early menopause should take HRT at least until fifty-one, the average age of menopause.

Surgical menopause (when the ovaries have been removed at operation), can cause symptoms to be particularly severe and distressing because of the sudden total loss of oestrogen (and decrease in testosterone).

When you are younger, your oestrogen requirements will be higher, so you may need a higher dose of oestrogen in HRT. In addition, younger women can also be more severely affected by the loss of testosterone, so you may need it earlier, and in higher doses (you'll find more advice on HRT in the next chapter).

Another option that younger women may prefer is the combined oral contraceptive pill, which contains both oestrogen and progesterone. There are some brands better suited to treating menopause than others, so please do discuss this with your doctor.

WHAT ABOUT FERTILITY?

There is roughly a 5–10 per cent chance of getting pregnant naturally following a POI diagnosis.[2] And as we get older, the chance of getting pregnant, along with the quality of our eggs, decreases and the risk of miscarriage goes up.

If you have POI and think you may want to have children now or in the future, make sure you get referred to a fertility specialist to talk about your options as soon as possible. The Daisy Network is an excellent charity which offers support to women with POI (www.daisynetwork.org.)

WHAT ABOUT CONTRACEPTION? DO I NEED IT?

Yes, if you still have ovaries and want to avoid getting pregnant, because HRT is not a form of contraception. Even women with a long-standing history of POI still need contraception if they want to be certain not to get pregnant.

HOW LONG TO TAKE IT FOR?

Typically, if you are under fifty, you should take it for two years after your last period. (When a woman is over fifty, it should be taken for one year after the last period.) It is slightly different in women with POI due to the small chance of ovulation and you should discuss this with your doctor.

Some good options are the Mirena coil, which can also act as the progesterone element of HRT, or a combined oral contraceptive pill, which has both oestrogen and progesterone. Over the age of fifty-five, a woman is no longer considered to be fertile and so you can cease to use contraception.

---

[2] L.M. Nelson, (2009), 'Clinical practice. primary ovarian insufficiency, *New England Journal of Medicine*, 360(6), pp.606-14, doi.org/10.1056/NEJMcp0808697

Over the last few years I feel like I've spoken to more and more women who have gone through an early menopause. Maybe it's just that more of us are talking about it, but weirdly it feels like it might be getting more common. It is often when women have been thrown into early menopause by treatment or an operation. Look, in some cases these women have received lots of support, and they have been offered that as a matter of course. But, sadly, it's sometimes left up to them to push for the help that they need, which is the last thing they want to do. And the last thing they feel able to do.

'Radiotherapy left me menopausal.' — Sima

Sima experienced menopause at the age of thirty-four, after having radiotherapy for Stage 3 bowel cancer.

I had every treatment to make me cancer-free but pelvic radiotherapy left me menopausal... the menopause devastated me. I have found it harder to come to terms with, and to get treatment for, than cancer. I have paid to see a specialist since 2019 and it has consequently been hugely improved by HRT.

Let that sink in for a moment: Sima found it harder to get treatment for menopause than treatment for *cancer*. That makes my blood boil.

And while it's brilliant to hear how well Sima is doing now, it's outrageous that she had to go private to get the help she deserved in the first place. You shouldn't have to, but if you are facing a similar situation to Sima, you need to inform yourself as much as possible. Don't be afraid to ask questions, push for what you deserve – answers, advice and treatment.

Before you go and talk to anybody, or before you speak to somebody on the phone, **write things down**, so that you are not stumbling for words in the appointment, and so you can be very clear and concise with your needs.

→ Can you explain my options to me?

→ What sort of care will I need going forward?

→ Should I be referred to a specialist?

Push, push, push for what you need to feel better again. It will be worth it in the end.

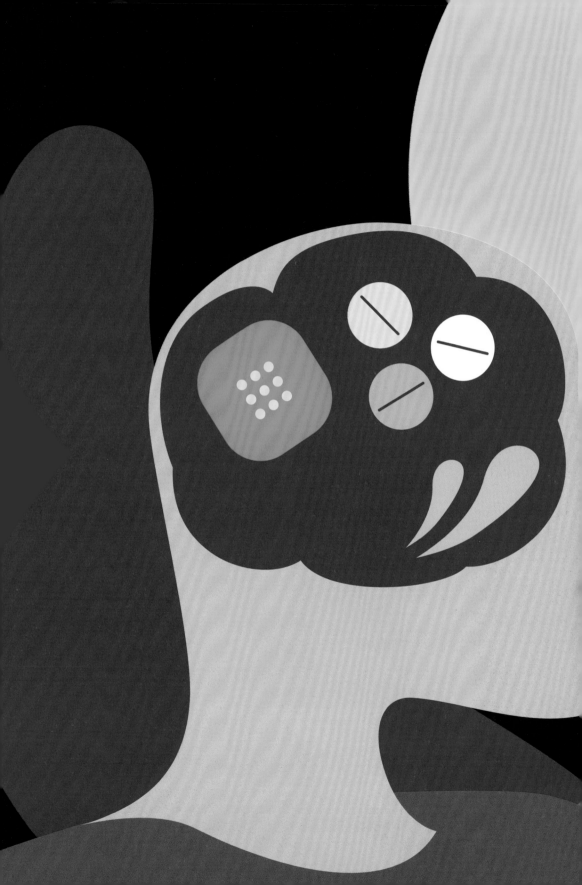

CHAPTER 5

NOW FOR THE SCIENCE BIT: HRT DEMYSTIFIED

HRT helped me rediscover myself.

I had disappeared, and now I'm back.

I want to demystify and de-demonise HRT so other women can rediscover themselves.

Just 1 in 10 of women who could benefit from HRT actually take it.[1]

HRT. Three tiny letters; one GIANT leap for womankind. And, in fact, mankind. And, in fact, allkind – childrenkind, everybodykind. Because when we're ok, everyone's ok.

Oh my God, I cannot tell you the difference that HRT has made to my life, and to the people, friends and family in my life. To my job, to my enjoyment – everything. It saved my career. It's just made me healthier – I can feel that – and generally more fun to be around.

Before I got on the HRT, I'd lost that sense of fun. I'd lost my essence. So I want all women who want and can have HRT to experience that same reawakening. I want them to experience that second spring that I've had since I started taking it. And as we've heard from many women through their own stories, sometimes it's a lifesaver. Literally.

Even though HRT has been available for half a century, so many of us just don't know enough about it (and I'm counting myself amongst that number, before I started on my menopausing crusade). I mean really, like, almost nothing. And 10 per cent of women who would benefit from it are actually taking it.[1]

That is such a tiny number, and I believe that is mostly because HRT is still considered 'bad' for us. For all the secrecy, shame and misinformation around it, you could be forgiven for thinking and believing that HRT is made from horse's wee, and that it's going to give you breast cancer, and it's so unnatural…

BUT YOU WOULD BE WRONG!

HRT is completely transformative. It does not just delay your menopause, it puts you back where you were. Hormone replacement therapy is exactly what it says; you aren't taking *more* hormones than you had before, you are merely replacing the ones that you are losing.

A lot of women that I meet tell me: 'Well, you know, I've got a few symptoms, I'm not sleeping that well and I've got a bit of brain fog, I'm weeing quite a lot in the night, I've got broken sleep and everything … I'm a bit ratty, but I think I'm just going to soldier on for another couple of years and sort of try to just, like, wait until I'm really bad, and then I'll take it.'

WHY?? Why are you doing that? You don't have to wait until you are on your knees before you ask your doctor for it. There are many, many signs pointing to the fact that if you start it early – when you get your first symptoms – there are good health benefits to it.

When it comes to the ingredients, and all the different ways that you can take HRT, there are so many different choices and so many combinations – all of it has come an incredibly long way in recent years.

---

[1] G.P Cumming, et al. (2015) 'The need to do better – Are we still letting our patients down and at what cost?', *Post Reproductive Health*, 21 (2), pp. 56–62. Doi.org/10.1177/2053369115586122

So what I need you to do is to have all the facts at your fingertips, so you can march – that's what I want you to do, MARCH! – head held high, shoulders back, waving a piece of paper with everything that you need written on it. Then you can go to your GP, and tell them what you *want* and what you *need*.

I want HRT to be as easy to get hold of as the pill. Women are started on the pill very freely, and it's less safe than HRT! We've all been taking that like they are just sweets for years.

So this chapter is all about getting under the skin of HRT. We're going to tell you what it's made from, how it works and why it doesn't just take care of your symptoms, it also takes care of your long-term health.

You can go for patches, you can have pills, stickies, sprays or choose oestrogen only (that's only if you don't have a womb anymore), and you can also go for combination, systemic, topical ... I mean, hello? The list of options is endless. But we've got Dr Naomi, so it's all going to be ok. She's going to be giving us a masterclass on the different ways that you can take HRT.

We're also going to be looking at how to deal with any side-effects that you might get in the first few months, which are very common and sometimes make women want to give up their HRT.

And we're going to be talking testosterone. It's been a dirty word,

and it's been something that women have been embarrassed to take, because we think it is not *our* hormone. But it is our hormone! Don't fear it, we are reclaiming it right here, right now!

We're going to take you through a little bit of a roadmap that you can follow to get to your praise-be moment. Yes! Hallelujah! We'll be able to tell you when you can start feeling like you again, which you all deserve.

I'm going to give you the lowdown on my own HRT regime, too, and give you some little tips and things that have helped me along the way. I hear from a lot of women that they've been told by their doctor that they have to come off HRT, and that obviously they can't take it forever so they're going to have to stop. We'll be answering that query, as well as why is your best mate on a higher dose than you? How do you stop the patch on your arse from falling off every time you sit down? (That's a really annoying one ... !)

We've been busy sifting through your stories. We've mined some late-night chats on social media, harnessed Dr Naomi's encyclopaedic knowledge and we have compiled a rock-solid list of HRT frequently asked questions that literally leaves no stone left unturned.

And we're going to be hearing about your ups and downs, success stories – and failures – about all things HRT.

HRT EXPLAINED;
BUT FIRST, A PEP TALK

'I had to give in.'

I never want to hear this in relation to menopause care. Look, if you're struggling and you are finding it really hard … in fact, no! Not even if you're finding it really hard; if you're just struggling a little bit, then you need and deserve help. And if that involves HRT, then that is IN NO WAY giving in.

Listen, I talk to women whose well-meaning friends or loved ones tell them that, you know, menopause is a *natural process*, and they should ('should' is a word bathed in shame) get through it without help.

'Well, you can only be on it for a few years.'

'Why would you want to put that poison in you?'

'HRT isn't natural.'

'Your symptoms will be worse when you come off that stuff.'

'You're only postponing the inevitable.'

Let's once and for all clear up the misconception that HRT is a last-resort treatment if you can't cope, or when symptoms get too bad. Look, think

about it for a second. If you were thyroid deficient (like I am), is taking thyroxine 'giving in'? No. If you are diabetic, is taking insulin 'giving in'? No. If you need oestrogen, is taking HRT the easy way out? NO. If you lack oestrogen, taking HRT is NOT GIVING IN. And no one – NO ONE – should ever make you feel embarrassed, ashamed or scared about opting for HRT.

As for the argument that HRT isn't natural – it's actually not natural for humans to get into a car or on an aeroplane. It's not natural for us to have antibiotics, blood transfusions or treatments for cancer. We humans weren't designed to live well into our eighties and nineties, but thankfully not being 'natural' doesn't stop us doing any of these things.

Knowing about HRT – what it is, what it does and what it doesn't do – is ESSENTIAL. Informing yourself will help you to make a choice that is completely yours. Empower yourself. This is your body, your life, your happiness.

'I'm starting to feel human again.' — Allison

Allison started taking HRT when she was forty-seven, but, like me, she kept quiet about it.

People might judge me, she thought, they'll see HRT as a bit of a cop out because they think it's a woman's right of passage just to suffer. When she turned fifty her GP took her off HRT but offered no alternative, so – boom! – there she was, back at square one.

Then in 2018 I started to feel a little better, and thought I was coming out the other side, but in December that year my beloved mum died, and literally overnight my symptoms came back.

By 2021, she was really sadly still struggling and gaining weight. She saw my *Sex, Myths and the Menopause* documentary and bravely decided then that she was going to call her GP.

I made a phone appointment, and as I was waiting for the call I was telling myself, whichever GP calls me, they are going to say I'm too old now to take it, or I'm too overweight, but when they did call they couldn't be more different.

Firstly, it was a female GP, secondly, she totally understood me. She also asked me if I'd watched Davina's documentary as she highly recommended it.

After a lengthy conversation she put me on the patch, and said she was surprised I wasn't offered it when I came off the tablets.

I've now been on the patch for just over a month, and my menopause symptoms are slowly easing. The weight is still an issue, but now I'm starting to feel human again I'll get motivated with diet and exercise.

Oh my god, reading Allison's story made me both happy and absolutely flipping furious at the same time. I'm so mad that she had to hide taking HRT, because she was scared of what other people thought of her.

I am furious she was taken off HRT with no explanation or alternative. And I am so pleased that she saw our doc, and she found a doctor who got her, and helped her.

'I honestly thought I was losing my mind.' — Dawn

Dawn had to wait three long years to find a doctor who would prescribe her HRT, after being told at forty-three that she was too young for perimenopause.

I went to see a private gynae who listened to everything I said, and she told me she could help me. I sat in her office and sobbed like a baby. She prescribed HRT and it honestly gave me my life back.

I'm 58 now and I don't ever plan to come off it – not if I can help it anyway. No woman should have to suffer the debilitating symptoms of menopause… NHS doctors need to be trained up on the treatment of the menopause.

Dawn saying that she has been given her life back is something I often hear, and I think that's because potentially people have been going through perimenopausal symptoms for a long time before they noticed it. So there is this sense of, *I feel better than I have done in years*. Because, possibly, you haven't actually felt yourself for years, and it's been a subtle decline. You suddenly have more energy and zest for life than you've ever had before.

All I want is for you to have options, and the right information so you can go to your doctor and feel confident and empowered to ask for the treatment you deserve.

So, what <u>exactly</u> is HRT? Is it really made from horses' wee?

The idea of replacing hormones during menopause has been around for longer than you probably think. Back in the 1940s, the Food and Drug Administration in America approved Premarin, an oestrogen product designed to treat hot flushes. And yes, it was made from horse urine. In fact, the name comes from PREgnant MARes' urine. However, the oestrogen we use now is practically identical to the oestrogen our bodies produce, and it's rare for Premarin to be prescribed these days – more on that a bit later on...

Back to the timeline: in 1965, hormone replacement therapy became available in the UK and women have been using it for half a century now. So, what is in HRT? Well, the clue is in the name – HRT replaces the hormones that are depleted during perimenopause and menopause. And that's what makes it an absolute game-changer: by replacing your hormones, your symptoms will get better, and you can get back to living the life you want.

HRT is only available on prescription and it will:

Nearly always contain oestrogen.

Often contain progesterone.

Sometimes contain testosterone.

If your HRT only contains oestrogen, it's known as **oestrogen-only HRT**. If your HRT contains oestrogen and progesterone it is called **combined HRT**. If you take oestrogen and progesterone every day it is called **continuous combined HRT** and if you take oestrogen every day but progesterone for only part of the month it is called **combined sequential HRT** or **cyclical HRT**.

WHY WOULD I TAKE ONE TYPE OVER THE OTHER?

Whether you take oestrogen on its own or oestrogen plus progesterone depends on whether you have a uterus (that is whether or not you have had a hysterectomy or not).

Taking oestrogen on its own without progesterone can overstimulate the lining of the womb, which is called the endometrium. If this was to continue over time, eventually it could lead to endometrial cancer. This risk is reduced by prescribing progesterone, or progestogen, as the synthetic version of progesterone is known.

Think of the endometrium as a patch of grass in your garden: if oestrogen is the sunshine and water that makes the grass and the rest of the garden grow, progesterone is the lawn mower that keeps it under control. Progesterone protects the endometrium, so the oestrogen can carry on bringing sunshine and water to the rest of your body.

You can have oestrogen-only HRT if you have had your uterus removed, but you should be prescribed combined HRT if:

→ You've had a partial or total hysterectomy. This is because some uterine lining may still remain.

→ You have a history of endometriosis. With endometriosis, the lining of the womb (the endometrium) can grow outside the uterus. So even if the uterus is removed at hysterectomy, endometrial tissue can remain and be stimulated by additional oestrogen. So it is important to take progesterone to prevent additional stimulation of the potential pockets of tissue. We'll be covering this later in the book in more detail (see page 256).

PATCHES, PILLS, GELS, SPRAYS... HOW DO I TAKE HRT?

Ok ladies, here comes the conundrum. Which one do you take?

Even after you've decided that HRT *is* for you, you've got some more big decisions to make, because there are dozens upon dozens of different combinations that you can take.

I was quite lucky because my body really got on well with the first treatment of oestrogen that I was put on; I was given a patch. Now, oestrogen patches are a postcode lottery. I am on Estradot – which is the smaller rectangular patch – and I put mine on my hip and am very lucky because I feel like it literally sticks like glue. The patch, it's important to say, is translucent. So it doesn't matter what colour skin you have, it will match the shade of your skin. I like the patch a lot because I just don't have to think about it. It works for me.

I can shower, I can swim, I can sweat, I can exercise. I can do everything and it never, ever comes off. I have heard that the larger patches are not as sticky, and it's for this reason – for the stickiness really, rather than anything else – that women find themselves changing over to gel sometimes. I was lucky with the stickers that I get in my area of the country – I live in the southeast of the UK – Estradot are good at sticking.

I was put on the progesterone pill, Utrogestan. Often women are put on Utrogestan and they take it at night because it gives them a slightly sedative effect. But it just didn't agree with me in terms of bleeding – I was bleeding all over the place, my periods were so irregular, and I felt a bit out of sorts. I had had the Mirena coil before, and I'd always thought that it hadn't agreed with me, but later realised I was probably just perimenopausal, even back then. And not in a good place. So I went back on the Mirena coil and I haven't looked back.

My HRT regime is the Mirena coil giving me slow-release progesterone, because I still have a womb, and I am on the 100 microgram patches of Estradot twice a week. I've had a couple of night sweats in the last year, so the day after that, and for a couple of days after, I've

maybe taken an extra pump of oestrogen gel on top. But generally, I don't really need the extra pump. I also take testosterone, but we'll talk about that later. It can all seem pretty bewildering, and I've got a girlfriend who has literally been trying to find the right combination for a year, but she hasn't given up. You might find that patches work better for you than a spray. Another girlfriend of mine feels great with three pumps of gel, but yet another girlfriend takes five, and she's like, 'Oh my God, I'm so sticky, I'd rather have a patch.' It is hard, I know, but don't give up. Concentrate on finding what works for you.

It's a bit of a minefield, but the variety and choice is actually a good thing. It means that you and your doctor can hit on the right regime for you, based on your needs, your lifestyle and your medical history.

And if things aren't working out as well as you'd like, or if you've still got symptoms, tweak it. There's a lot of tweaking to be done when you start taking HRT, or when you move from perimenopause to menopause. It is relatively straightforward to switch your method and alter your dose. The last thing you want to do is come off HRT altogether without exploring ALL of your options first.

THE OESTROGEN ELEMENT OF HRT – PUTTING THE GOOD STUFF BACK IN

There are lots of different ways you can take the oestrogen part of your HRT. Deciding which one to start with should begin with a conversation with your doctor about your lifestyle, health background and personal preference. Let's take a closer look into the different types – how you use them, when you use them, and the various pros and cons of each – so you can be the judge of what might work for you.

I'm going to leave you in Dr Naomi's expert hands to take you through everything you need to know about the different types of HRT.

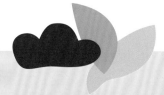

DR NAOMI'S HRT MASTERCLASS PART 1: OESTROGEN

When you replace oestrogen, whatever method you choose will deliver oestrogen to you daily. The most commonly used oestrogen these days is called 17-beta estradiol. This is a body-identical hormone, which means it has the same structure as the oestrogen made by your body. Oestrogen can either be given transdermally (through the skin) or orally (by mouth). How well one method works over the other will depend on how well your skin absorbs oestrogen. Unfortunately, there is no real way of knowing about absorption in advance, so the first few months can be a case of trial and error. But be patient, trust the process. You will get there.

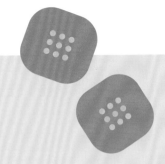

TRANSDERMAL OESTROGEN:

This is oestrogen that is delivered via the skin in the form of a patch, gel or spray. Unlike when you take oral oestrogen, transdermal HRT bypasses your liver and there is no increased risk of blood clots, stroke or gallbladder disease.

PATCHES

A patch will contain oestrogen which is absorbed through the skin and sometimes is combined with progesterone. The oestrogen-only patches come in a variety of strengths. They are small, thin plastic squares that stick to the skin.

Pros

+ Patches are clear, so they are suitable for all skin colours.

+ It's a discreet method, as you can fit them underneath a bikini or swimsuit.

+ They are convenient if you are short on time.

+ They come in different sizes and doses – starting at 25 micrograms and working up to 100 micrograms, so they can be a good option if you need higher doses.

How do I use them?

Peel off the foil backing and stick the patch on your bottom, thigh or upper leg. It releases a steady dose of oestrogen and normally needs replacing twice a week.

Cons

– Some women find the patches are hard to keep in place, especially if they have oily skin. They might come off in the shower, or the edges start to curl. They can be unpleasant to remove.

– If you opt for a patch you are committing to a set dose, so it can be harder to adjust the dose if you need to. In some circumstances, you *can* cut the patches up to have a smaller dose, but you should only do this under the direction of your doctor.

– Some women don't like the fact that they are partially visible.

GEL

There are two types of gel available in the UK: a pump bottle or a sachet called Sandrena. The pump bottle, known as Oestrogel, is widely available on the NHS and it is very cost-effective, so there's no reason why it can't be an option. There are also versions available in Australia, Canada and the US.

How do I use it?

With Oestrogel, you push the top of the dispenser down and it releases a 'pump' or little blob of gel. You spread the gel as thinly as possible on the inside and outside of your arm from your wrist to your shoulder, but you can also put it on thighs, tops of legs, bottom, inner thighs – just make sure you avoid the breast area.

Pros

+ Like the patches, this is transdermal so it bypasses the liver.

+ Gel absorbs well into the skin.

+ It is convenient because you can use tiny doses, so if you are hormone-sensitive you can start with a small dose and build it up.

+ Some women prefer the convenience of sachets when travelling.

Cons

– If you are using a higher dose you'll need copious amounts – four pumps doesn't sound like much but it is enough to cover all four limbs.

– Some women don't like the sticky, cold feeling of applying gel, especially in winter.

– The sachets can be messy and less precise than a measured pump and create more waste.

– You need to give it time to dry so it won't rub off on your clothes, and remember to wash your hands afterwards to avoid rubbing it onto your kids, partners or pets.

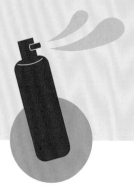

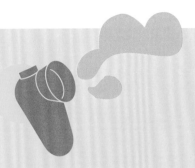

SPRAY

The spray is called Lenzetto and is one of the newest products, launched in the UK in 2020, but it is starting to become more readily available. It can now be accessed in countries across Europe, the USA and Australia.

How do I use it?

Take off the plastic cover, hold the bottle upright and rest the plastic cone flat against your skin (a lot of women use the spray along their inner forearm, or inner thigh). Press the pump to release one spray; if your prescription calls for more than one spray, move it further down the arm or thigh for each additional spray.

You'll need to let the spray air dry for about an hour before allowing clothing to touch it, and wait at least another hour before showering or swimming.

Pros

+ Like gel and patches, the spray is transdermal.

+ Quick application and dries quickly.

+ Less copious and less of an alcohol smell compared to the gel.

+ The dose is easy to increase or decrease.

Cons

− It can be harder to get it prescribed on the NHS.

− It can require quite a few sprays to eliminate symptoms.

− You need to let it dry before clothing can touch it.

SYSTEMIC OESTROGEN:

ORAL TABLET

When women start HRT they are often prescribed oestrogen in tablet form. It is often combined with progesterone. There is a new product called Bijuve, which is a body-identical oestrogen and progesterone in one tablet. It is suitable for post-menopausal women.

How do I use it?

Take one tablet daily.

Pros

+ A pill can be convenient if you are used to taking a tablet daily, for example the contraceptive pill, and you like that kind of familiar routine.

+ If you have skin sensitivity an oral tablet could be beneficial, as it might be harder for you to find a transdermal (through the skin) product that you aren't allergic or sensitive to.

+ It can be an easy way of taking both oestrogen and progesterone together.

Cons

− Taking an oral version of oestrogen slightly increases your risk of a blood clot, stroke and gallbladder disease.

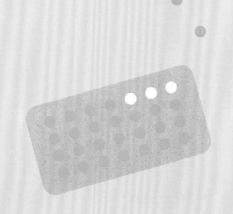

VAGINAL OESTROGEN:

Vaginal dryness and urinary symptoms can be a huge issue during perimenopause and menopause. Thinning tissues can lead to itching, soreness and painful sex, but also urinary symptoms such as going more often, getting up at night and leakage as well as recurrent urinary tract infections. When systemic HRT (in the form of a gel patch, spray or tablet) puts back the oestrogen, this can help the genital tissues become soft and supple again, but about one in three women will need something extra: topical oestrogen.

Topical oestrogen includes creams, rings and pessaries that you insert inside your vagina or apply to your vulva. Oestrogen can then act directly on local tissues but because it is minimally absorbed, there is practically no risk. We'll be looking at topical oestrogen in much more detail in the Dry Vagina Monologues chapter.

DR NAOMI'S MASTERCLASS PART 2: NOW FOR THE PROGESTERONE BIT

If you take oestrogen and you have a uterus you will need to take progesterone, too. Two of the best options are micronised progesterone (Utrogestan, Cyclogest and Lutigest) and the Mirena coil.

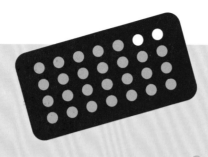

MICRONISED PROGESTERONE

Micronised progesterone is the most body-similar progesterone available. This means it has practically the same chemical structure as the progesterone in our bodies.

Pros

+   This is the safest progesterone for breasts.

+   It is body identical – it has the same chemical structure as the progesterone in your body.

+   It has fewer side-effects than older types of progestogen.

+   Has a sedative effect – so it is recommended you take it at nighttime.

How do I use it?

If you are post-menopausal you take an oral tablet daily. If you are in the perimenopause you take an oral tablet for part of the month as a cycle. It is sometimes prescribed by specialists off-licence to be used vaginally if you have progesterone-type side-effects.

Cons

-   Bleeding can be a side-effect in the first few months.

-   Some women – particularly those who have had PMS in the past – can be particularly sensitive to progesterone. It can trigger PMS-type symptoms like anger, rage, tearfulness, breast tenderness and bloating. If you experience these symptoms, please speak to your doctor about changing your dose or the method of delivering it.

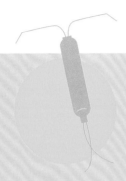

MIRENA COIL

A Mirena coil is a soft, flexible, T-shaped device which releases progestogen at a slow and steady rate. It can be used as the endometriol protection component of HRT. It can stay in place for up to five years. It's an excellent option if you are looking to combine your HRT with a contraceptive.

Pros

+ It helps control bleeding.

+ It acts as a contraceptive.

+ It releases a steady amount of progesterone that is minimally absorbed, so it is a good option if you are sensitive to progesterone.

+ It stays in place for five years, so you don't have to remember to take tablets.

How do I use it?

This must be fitted by a doctor or nurse. It takes about twenty minutes to fit, and is inserted into the uterus. Once fitted, you should not be able to feel it.

Cons

− While the vast majority of women have a coil fitted without pain or side-effects, for some women, fitting can be uncomfortable. If you experience discomfort, please ask your practitioner to stop. To reduce discomfort take some paracetamol beforehand. Book the afternoon off work to rest after it is fitted.

TESTOSTERONE: WHY WE NEED TO RECLAIM IT

Ok, I want to ask you something. What comes to mind when you hear the word 'testosterone'?

For me, it's man, muscles, moustaches, hairy chests, protein shakes, chowing down on man-sized protein bars, and comparing quads and biceps in a steam room. I'm also thinking, guys shouting each other down, cavemen, protruding foreheads and dick-swinging.

But no! NO NO NO. Not. Even. Close. Guess what? I mean, this blew me away as well, right: testosterone is a female hormone. We actually produce it in our ovaries and other parts of our bodies, too. (God, we are SO clever.)

HRT has helped me massively, but when I first started taking it, I've got to say that I still felt like there was something missing. As if I was better, my symptoms were better – the massively debilitating ones like lack of sleep, night sweats, that kind of rage – all of those were better, but I still wasn't firing on all cylinders; I still wasn't quite me.

I was prescribed testosterone by my private gynaecologist. I feel terrible that I can afford to go to a private gynaecologist about this stuff while it's not available widely on the NHS, but we really are trying

to change that. And that's why I'm talking about it and I'm working with Carolyn Harris MP and so many other badass menopause warriors to try to change this.

I really can, hand on heart, tell you it's been a game-changer for me. My mood, libido, memory, general ability to cope with whatever life throws at me, have all come back. When I walk into a meeting I feel like I am on it. I feel like I have ideas. I feel that my brain is firing on all cylinders.

So if it's such good stuff, then why on earth aren't more of us taking it? Well, that's because testosterone isn't licensed on the NHS. So what does that mean? Is it because it's too expensive? No. Is it because it's unsafe? No.

The only types of testosterone products available on the NHS are gels or creams, and they're designed to be used by men. And because these products are not licensed to be used by women, GPs will only prescribe them if they are comfortable to do so off licence. Which, understandably, not all GPs are.

Excuse me? That's OUTRAGEOUS, right? It's my next big focus in the fight for better menopause care, it really is, and it's something all of you out there are asking about. So, what's the score?

Testosterone is a female hormone – we actually produce more testosterone than oestrogen.[2] When testosterone levels fall during perimenopause and menopause, it can manifest as loss of libido, strength, power, get up and go, and brain sharpness. Replacing it as part of HRT can be the final piece of the jigsaw.

Guidance from the British Menopause Society is that: if a woman has been adequately re-oestrogenised with HRT but her symptoms have not completely resolved, especially if she has a symptom of low libido, then testosterone replacement should be considered.

Testosterone levels can easily be calculated with a simple blood test called an FAI (Free Androgen Index) to assess whether a woman is low in available testosterone. Using this test in conjunction with assessing symptoms, it can be relatively straightforward to decide if you need testosterone.

Women with a history of POI, early menopause or surgical menopause, in particular, can feel the effects of low testosterone the most.

Because the only available products on the NHS are unlicensed, some GPs are understandably reluctant to prescribe it. If you feel you would benefit from testosterone, ask to be referred to a specialist clinic.

Another option – and I know it's not available to everyone – is to see someone privately. Private clinics are willing to prescribe a testosterone cream called AndroFeme, which is imported from Australia and is designed to be used by women. My dream is that no woman would have to go to a private clinic to get prescribed testosterone. It feels completely unfair and outrageous that that concept is even something that I had to write about and it isn't the case in every country. But hopefully in a year's time, or two years' time, I will be rewriting this chapter and taking that bit out.

[2] British Menopause Society (2022), 'Testosterone replacement in menopause' https://thebms.org.uk/publications/tools-for-clinicians/testosterone-replacement-in-menopause/

WHEN WILL I START TO FEEL LIKE ME AGAIN?

I've got to say that I was one of the lucky ones because, as I said earlier, I did manage to get onto a regime that suited me pretty quickly, after a little hiccup with the progesterone, but the minute I got the Mirena coil (maybe six months into my journey) I felt fantastic. And a year after that, when I started taking testosterone, that was it. Done. And I'm still on the same regime now.

When I started taking oestrogen, even though my periods were all over the place, my symptoms and my brain fog lifted – I would say within a few days. Some people say it takes a few weeks, but my night sweats finished in three or four days. I can remember waking up in dry sheets, having slept for a whole night without going to the loo – it was extraordinary.

'I feel happier, more positive and much more in control.' — Annabel

There are stories of when women get the ta-da moment of thinking to themselves, *I'm back* ... One of the ones that really moved me was when a woman was talking about feeling joy again, laughing with her daughter about something – and she hadn't done that for years. Then there are women like Annabel, who tried pretty much every herbal remedy before starting HRT.

I turned fifty this year but have been suffering with perimenopausal symptoms for the last couple of years with HORRENDOUS hot flushes. At first I thought I could handle it but it became just too much to bear so I made an appointment to see my GP.

Unfortunately, she was very much against HRT because of the increased risk of cancer, so she sent me away with a list of natural treatments like sage, red clover, etc. I even gave up my beloved caffeine!

I tried for a good ten months but no change. After watching Davina's programme, I made an appointment with a different GP at my practice who initially discouraged me again because of the risk of cancer.

I was persistent and she was going to prescribe tablets but, again, because of Davina's programme I was armed with the knowledge that there are patches or creams available, so asked for one of those instead.

I am now on week four of HRT patches and the hot flushes have just started to ease, I feel happier, more positive and much more in control.

Boom! Mic-drop. We are all different, it is not one size fits all. For some it is four days and you feel better, for others it can take months. I am just so glad that you are feeling better, Annabel.

As I said, I was lucky in that my symptoms improved pretty quickly, but I know not everyone has the same experience. Don't lose heart, though: remember, it can take a while to hit on a routine that works for you. This can mean dose changes and adjustments, but please don't give up.

Every woman's experience of taking HRT is different, but as a guide this is when you can expect to feel better once you start taking HRT.

1 week–1 month

Symptoms such as hot flushes and night sweats can start to ease off within a couple of weeks. You may feel like any anxiety is starting to lift.

1 month–3 months

Mood issues, aches, pains and skin-related symptoms may improve.

Vaginal dryness and urinary symptoms can also resolve within a few months. If they don't, please ask your doctor about the possibility of using vaginal oestrogen (see page 127).

Up to 1 year

Libido can be one of the last things to come back.

The perimenopause can be a moving target because there will still be your own hormone production carrying on in the background.

LET'S TALK ABOUT SIDE-EFFECTS

Short-term side-effects from oestrogen can include breast tenderness or nausea. Starting on oestrogen can also lead to some irregular, and sometimes heavy, bleeding. This can last for about three to six months.

Some women can really struggle with the side-effects from progesterone, particularly those who already suffer from PMS. Side-effects can include breast tenderness, anger, rage, tearfulness and bloating, puffiness or swelling, and gastric symptoms such as acid reflux. If this is the case, please discuss with your doctor other ways that you could take progesterone.

POTENTIAL RED FLAGS

Should you experience any of the following symptoms, please discuss with your doctor urgently:

→ Any new bleeding (unless you have just started HRT or have just increased the dose) or heavy or unexplained bleeding that lasts for three to six months.

→ Any pain in your calves, or shortness of breath, as this could be a sign of a clot. Oral oestrogen can slightly increase the risk of clots.

→ Itching, swelling and shortness of breath could be a sign of an allergic reaction.

→ Breast swelling, lumps or tenderness, particularly if it is on one side only.

MAKING IT STICK: HOW I USE MY HRT

So you've just left the chemist, you're clutching a paper bag, you've got pills, patches, gels, sprays, advice from your doctor ringing in your ears. Oh my goodness, what do you do now?

So the first thing you need to do is find a routine that you can stick to. I've just changed mine, actually, and I think I'm a lot more efficient now. I do it this way: I put all of my hormones next to my toothbrush, because I know that I brush my teeth twice a day. I'm usually a bath-at-night person, but sometimes I also have a shower in the morning if I need to wash my hair, and I will do that before I apply anything, obviously, because otherwise you wash off all your hormones. I get out of the shower and apply my patch if I'm doing that (on a Monday or a Thursday) and I then get my pea-sized bit of testosterone and rub it onto my thigh. I then wash my hands. Sometimes, if I've had a night sweat or whatever and I need a pump of gel, I'll do that and rub it in on the top of my arm like a moisturiser and I just leave it there. Then I brush my teeth. And I brush them for two minutes, which means that the gel has completely soaked in in those two minutes. Then I put my clothes on, and I take my thyroxine.

I mean, I'm rattling. Literally. All those medicines in the morning.

What your doctor will generally say is, if you're going to put on the gel or spray, leave it to dry fully before you get dressed. But with the gel, leave it for a few hours before you're going to go for a shower or swim (that's why I put it on after the shower in the morning).

If you have got a patch that's falling off, I would try putting them in different places, because sometimes, if I put it too far round the back it comes off easily. It's just a case of where is the best place on your hips to put the sticker. Even if you move it one or two centimetres in another direction, it might not fall off as much.

I started off on 100 micrograms of Estradot twice a week. I was given that dose straight off the bat and it really worked for me. But sometimes you need to have your dosage upped quite a lot, because most people, I think, who go to a GP get prescribed 25 micrograms, and that is quite a low dosage. But it is a good idea to start low because you do sometimes need to work up to a higher dose with oestrogen – you don't want to suddenly go in for a big hit. Taking 100 micrograms of Estradot twice a week is a good amount, and it works really nicely for me.

As I've said quite a lot, I use the Mirena coil for my progesterone. It's slow-release, so no more periods, I can just forget about it. I've basically had a Mirena coil for fifteen years (obviously not the same one, I've had a new one every five years). If you don't have a coil but you still need progesterone you can take Utrogestan, which is a tablet. This is the kind of gold-standard progesterone: it's body identical, you can take it at night, and it's even got a slightly, kind of lovely, sleepy side-effect that can help you sleep.

Then, as we've talked about before, there's the testosterone cream. I have used Androfeme, but actually the gynaecologist that I see prescribes me a man's Testogel, which comes in a little sachet and you put a tiny, weeny amount – like a tenth of the sachet – on every day. With Androfeme you need a pea-sized amount but if you're using men's Testogel you have to use, obviously, a much smaller dose than a man would use, between a seventh and a tenth of that quantity. Try not to think about your HRT in terms of the number of micrograms, pumps, sprays or doses, and instead ask 'is it helping me?' If the answer is yes, then it is the right dose for you. If not, please talk to your doctor.

DR NAOMI: WHEN HRT IS NOT GOING WELL

I'VE STARTED HRT AND IT'S NOT WORKING. WHAT NOW?

Doctors are taught to give the lowest effective amount of any medication. You may find your doctor or menopause specialist starts you on a lower dose, anticipating they may well need to increase it at a later date. Women absorb HRT in different ways and they respond to hormones in different ways, too. Some women will absorb them well, others less so. Doses of all hormones can require adjusting – both to increase and decrease them. If you don't feel like the HRT is having an effect, your doctor might look at increasing it. Please discuss with them.

I'M GETTING SIDE-EFFECTS. WHAT NOW?

If you are experiencing side-effects most of the time these will settle, especially breast tenderness, bleeding and nausea. If they persist beyond a couple of months, or become disruptive or uncomfortable please discuss with your doctor.

MY PMS HAS GOT WORSE SINCE I STARTED HRT. WHAT CAN I DO?

It may be that you are progesterone sensitive and that an alternative method or reduced dose might be suitable for you. The Mirena coil releases progesterone that is minimally absorbed and could be a better option. Alternatively you could trial a different progesterone or have a reduced dose under the care of your specialist.

DOES A HIGHER DOSE OF HRT MEAN IT IS LESS 'SAFE'

Some women will require higher doses to control their symptoms, particularly if they have had an early or surgically induced menopause.

It's natural to be concerned about having a higher dose, but if symptoms persist this indicates that your hormone levels have not been replaced sufficiently.

'Don't give up – kick menopause's ass!' — Helen

I was thirty-nine, bubbly, outgoing and life and soul of the party. Three years on, I was a mess. Tired, sore, grumpy and a shadow of the former me … what happened? Bloody hormones!

I developed crippling health anxiety out of nowhere and I tried everything; acupuncture, hypnotherapy, yoga, supplements and A LOT of horrible, horrible therapy, over a year of weekly sessions, and what cured me? HRT!

My GP didn't mention it, my smear nurse never mentioned it, not even Google thought to offer me a perimenopause diagnosis. A friend casually mentioned it and – eureka! – I was cured. Except it's not that easy!

The GP (after some begging) ran a blood test that suggested I wasn't perimenopausal, and I was floored, I was so convinced that perimenopause fitted my symptoms.

So I advocated for myself, withdrew savings and saw a specialist – and the rest is history. Why did I have to do that? Pay for it? Advocate for myself? Become my own bloody doctor, for crying out loud?! If I told my husband his penis would drop off at age forty, you can guarantee something would be done.

I cannot stress this enough, I WAS A BROKEN WOMAN AND NO ONE HELPED ME, EXCEPT ME!

So please, learn a lesson from me and don't waste months of your life discussing your abandonment issues with a therapist, your only abandonment issue is that your hormones have fucked off!

You can still have periods, the list of symptoms are mental, hot flushes don't always happen, your vajayjay doesn't always dry up, your sleep isn't always affected. Are you getting the idea that there's no 'normal' where menopause is concerned?

So read this book, read all the books, get informed, don't give up – and kick menopause's ass!

Yes, Helen! That's what I like! You are a menopause warrior, and you're so right. Read all the books, get informed and don't give up.

I'M ON HRT AND SOME OF MY SYMPTOMS HAVE STARTED COMING BACK. WHAT'S GOING ON?

When some women start HRT, there can be a 'honeymoon effect' where symptoms can resolve very quickly. However, this effect can wear off. This can be for multiple reasons; if you are perimenopausal, your initial HRT can work perfectly well at giving you a top-up, but as you move into menopause your body requires more. It can also happen to older women who have been on HRT for some time.

WHY DOES MY PATCH KEEP COMING OFF?

Some women find patches stick easier than others and this can depend on skin type, with patches sticking less well onto oily skin. Activities such as extended swimming or baths, saunas and steam rooms can impact on how long your patch will stick. If you are having trouble keeping a patch on, try adjusting where you stick it. But if you find these changes make no difference, you may benefit from changing the product you are using.

Some women find the patches can irritate their skin. You may find using one of the smaller patches better and rotating where you apply it.

I'M AWAY WITH GIRLFRIENDS AND I'VE FORGOTTEN MY HRT. CAN I JUST USE THEIRS INSTEAD?

No, everyone's prescription is individual to them, as is yours. If you have forgotten your HRT you can sometimes obtain an emergency prescription from a local pharmacy.

I'VE GOT AN OPERATION COMING UP. DO I NEED TO STOP TAKING MY HRT?

You might be asked to stop taking certain medications ahead of an operation to reduce the risk of complications like blood clots, but if you are using transdermal HRT, there is not usually a reason to stop taking it as this method does not increase the risk of clots. If you are taking oral oestrogen, it will depend on the type of surgery – for example, surgery involving arteries, veins, heart or lower parts of the body, increases the risk of clots. Please discuss this with your doctor.

If you are on oral HRT and you are going to have an operation that puts you at risk of clots, then your doctor could switch you onto transdermal HRT well in advance of the operation. Please discuss this with them.

CAN I RECYCLE MY HRT?

We should all be doing our bit to be greener, but medication is a bit of a grey area. Take your empty sachets, bottles and tubes back to your local pharmacy or chemist where they will dispose of them safely, and never flush medicines down the toilet.

You can put cardboard boxes that house your patches, sprays, gel bottles or pill blister packs in the recycling, as well as any patient information leaflets. Medicine blister packs can be recycled at pharmacies that are participating in the TerraCycle Medicine Packet Recycling Programme.[3] If you live in Australia, the Return Unwanted Medicines project is a national scheme where you can return out-of-date and unwanted medicines to pharmacies (www.returnmed.com.au). And if you live in the USA, the DEA (Drug Enforcement Administration) oversees a twice-yearly programme that allows you to drop off unwanted medicines safely (www.dea.gov/takebackday).

I'M IN MY 70S, CAN I START TAKING HRT FOR THE FIRST TIME?

There is a 'window of opportunity' from a woman's last period to when you would normally start HRT and consider it to be protective. This is because oestrogen has a positive effect on blood vessels and keeps them soft, supple, flexible and clean. After a period of time when there hasn't been any oestrogen, the vessels can become more furry and rigid, and it is thought at this point that taking oestrogen can become more risky.

After this time, the benefits are less clear, but it is never a blanket no. Please discuss this with your doctor and they will balance your individual risk and the benefits.

[3] Recycle Now, 'What to do with Medicines', www.recyclenow.com/what-to-do-with/medicines-0

CAN I STAY ON HRT FOREVER?

The answer is potentially, yes. As long as the benefits outweigh the risks, you can stay on it long term – in some women, this means forever.

While we don't yet have study data of women who have been on body-identical HRT for thirty or forty years, what we do know is that modern HRT is safe and it is protective.

Women feel good on HRT: it eases symptoms, protects long-term health in many ways and they enjoy living their lives on it – and that must count for a lot.

I WANT TO STOP TAKING HRT, HOW DO I GO ABOUT IT?

This really depends on why you want to come off it in the first place. If it's the case that you are suffering side-effects, your symptoms aren't getting better or are worsening, or you just aren't getting on with the method you are using, please speak to your doctor first. They should be looking at how to adjust your HRT to allow you to carry on.

Ultimately it is your body, and your decision, so if you still really want to come off HRT, do it under the supervision of a doctor.

Unless you are on a very low dose, stopping suddenly isn't the best idea. It's better to reduce your dose gradually to avoid a hormonal crash. If you change your mind, you can ask for the dosage to be increased again.

The only time you would be coming off HRT straight away is if you have had a diagnosis that suggests you shouldn't be on it.

AND FINALLY...
A MESSAGE OF HOPE

I wanted to share this story with you in full because it honestly made me want to punch the air when I read it. If you are struggling right now for whatever reason – job, family, divorce, whatever – I hope this story will light up even the smallest glimmer of hope that things can and will get better.

'I feel powerful and I feel like I am on this journey with an army of powerful women.' — Hayley

Over to you, Hayley...

Going through divorce was hard, so was supporting my children through this. But to start at forty-two to feel like I wasn't myself was the hardest thing of all. I remember the day that the anxiety, tension, anger, sadness and panic took hold. I stood in my kitchen after a day out with the kids, and I feel like I didn't stop crying for two years. Anxiety was my first symptom and it changed me. Night sweats, chronic tension, panic attacks all followed, and the crying just became my thing. You can blame divorce, work, stress, midlife challenges, but I knew this was more, I just didn't feel like me and it was terrifying.

I researched, over-shared with family and friends, cried some more. I took up meditation, it is a life-saver and my goodness it works in such profound ways, but it didn't resolve it all. I tried CBT, which helped so much, and I started to run – running for my head not my body was a totally different ball game, it was essential, so essential at times. I was open with my beautiful children, I didn't want them to be scared, they knew this was not Mummy and it was the menopause making me struggle, but it wouldn't beat me and I made sure they knew that.

Lots of listening to more powerful and knowledgeable women than me, they became my best friends – Dr Potter, Dr Newson, Davina, Lisa Snowdon, Meg Mathews, they didn't know me, but they knew what I was experiencing.

I felt slowly but surely that there was help out there. Three GP visits later and offers of antidepressants, I became another woman not being taken seriously. So, my lovely supportive partner found a menopause clinic, after all the learning he said it's time to not be afraid and to see if HRT is the answer or the support you need. I have been prescribed HRT and I am one day in. Last night I lay in bed a few hours after taking it. I felt euphoric, I felt like a child with fire in my belly. Too soon, I thought, but who knows, maybe this is my body breathing a sigh of relief and saying thank you.

I have no idea how this story ends, but I feel powerful and I feel like I am on this journey with an army of powerful women. And my young son said to me, 'Mummy, have you got the oestrogen now?' I said yes, and he cheered.

That is amazing.

THE BENEFITS OF HRT

Addressing troublesome menopause symptoms is only part of the story when it comes to HRT; it also has some really important protective qualities that can be overlooked in the conversations around symptoms, patches, coils and routines. For me, the long-term benefits are just as important as getting rid of the symptoms.

BONE HEALTH

When taken at the start of menopause, HRT can help prevent bone loss.[4] It is especially important if you have an early menopause or POI, but it can protect women of any age.

Some studies have shown that HRT can increase bone density by around five per cent in two years, and that it can reduce the risk of spinal and hip fractures by forty per cent.[4]

HEART HEALTH

Studies show that HRT may actually reduce your risk of heart disease if started before the age of sixty or within ten years of your menopause.[5] Coronary heart disease kills more than twice as many women as breast cancer in the UK every year, and it is the single biggest killer of women worldwide.[6]

METABOLIC HEALTH

There is evidence that oestrogen keeps fat distribution peripherally, which is healthier than being around the trunk. It may also have a beneficial effect on cholesterol[7] and sugar metabolism.[8]

SKIN HEALTH

Oestrogen helps maintain collagen structure, skin hydration, elasticity and

---

[4] Australasian Menopause Society (2018), 'Osteoporosis', www.menopause.org.au/hp/information-sheets/osteoporosis

[5] National Institute for Health and Care Excellence (2015), 'Menopause: Diagnosis and Management', www.nice.org.uk/guidance/ng23

[6] British Heart Foundation, 'Women and heart attacks', www.bhf.org.uk/informationsupport/conditions/heart-attack/women-and-heart-attacks

[7] M A Denke (1995) 'Effects of continuous combined hormone-replacement therapy on lipid levels in hypercholesterolemic postmenopausal women'.

[8] Espeland MA, Hogan PE, Fineberg SE, Howard G, Schrott H, Waclawiw MA, Bush TL (1998). 'Effect of postmenopausal hormone therapy on glucose and insulin concentrations'. PEPI Investigators, Diabetes Care

skin integrity. Hormone replacement therapy (HRT) has been shown to increase epidermal hydration, skin elasticity, skin thickness[9], and also reduces skin wrinkles.[10] Furthermore, the content and quality of collagen and the level of vascularization is enhanced.[11]

BRAIN HEALTH

Currently, the effect of HRT on the risk of dementia isn't very clear – some studies have found women who take HRT have a reduced risk of dementia, while others have contradicted this.

However, a 2021 study involving more than 600,000 women over three decades concluded that HRT is not linked to an *increased* risk of dementia.[12]

A 2022 study from the US reported that taking HRT for six years or more substantially decreases your risk of Alzheimer's and dementia, and many other neurological illnesses. In fact, women who underwent menopausal hormone therapy for six or more years were seventy-nine per cent less likely to develop Alzheimer's and seventy-seven per cent less likely to develop any neurodegenerative disease.[13]

Clearly much more research is needed into the area.

[9] Sator et al. (2001) 'The influence of hormone replacement therapy on skin ageing.' University of Vienna, Austria.

[10] Phillips et al. (2001) 'Hormonal effects on skin aging'. Clinics in Geriatric Medicine.

[11] Brincat et al. (1987) 'Skin collagen changes in post-menopausal women receiving different regimens of estrogen therapy.' Obstetrics & Gynecology.

[12] Y. Vinogradova et al. (2021),' Use of menopausal hormone therapy and risk of dementia: nested case-control studies using QResearch and CPRD databases', British Medical Journal, doi.org/10.1136/bmj.n2182

[13] Yu Jin Kim & Maira Soto et al. (2022) 'Association between menopausal hormone therapy and risk of neurodegenerative diseases' Center for Innovation in Brain Science, University of Arizona, Tucson.

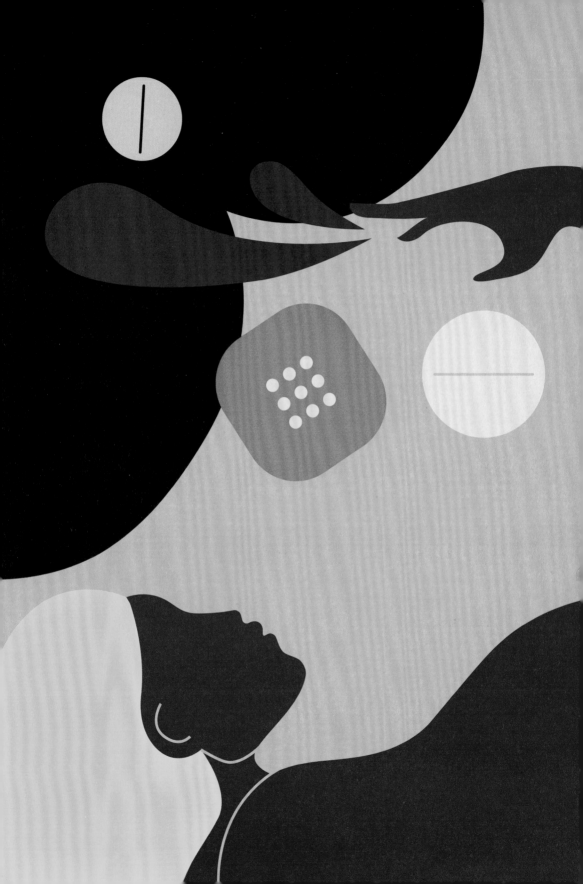

CHAPTER 6

HRT:
DEBUNKING
THE MYTHS

In my life, I try to basically be fairly straight up and straightforward. I am very honest with my feelings. I'm not a buttoned-up person. I will give you an uncomfortably long hug after I've only met you once; I talk to every single baby in the street; I have to talk to every person that walks past me with a dog, about their dog, and how old it is, and so on. I'm very social and I literally pour out my soul to anybody I ever meet in the ladies' loo in a nightclub. I'm very open.

But here's the weird thing. When I went on HRT, I felt SO ashamed, and it's hard to find the words to describe why I felt unable to tell friends. I think it was caught up in: I was old, I felt dried up, I felt ashamed that I couldn't grin and bear it when I was so tough – I'd had three home births, I had done this crazy Sport Relief challenge, but perimenopause floored me. And there I was, 'taking a drug' to make me feel better.

That's how I perceived it. I had friends of mine who all seemed so happy in their lives, coping with everything, so able. I just felt like I couldn't talk to them about it.

I really believed people would think that my decision to take HRT would be based in some sort of vanity – that I wanted to appear or look or feel younger, that in some way what I was doing was anti-natural. And I'd been so pro-natural up until that point: a drug-free birth, a clean-living lifestyle, exercise. I eat healthily. I felt like HRT was somehow negating all of those healthy lifestyle decisions that I was making.

It's so interesting what's happened to my perception of my hormones in recent years. I was helped to reframe the way that I look at it – and that is, hormone replacement therapy is exactly that. I am not trying to turn into a superhuman, to be able to lift weights suddenly or be able to do some extraordinary feat of sporting prowess. I'm not looking to become a nymphomaniac (although that would be nice?!). I'm not doing it to be thin, and I'm not doing it to make my face look younger. I'm doing it because my world was falling apart, and it helped me.

But now – and this is a very different spin on it – I'm actually taking it for the health benefits as well. Obviously, the relief from the symptoms is massive, but I am doing it because I am informed. I mean, I am REALLY informed. I have gone forensic on the menopause. I read SO many papers and resources, on everything – even parts of the menopause that don't affect me personally.

I am a massive advocate of freedom of choice; so whatever choice you make, it just has to be an informed one. So many women – too many women – are robbed of making that informed choice because of an absolutely unacceptable lack of available facts and an all-pervading mistrust of HRT.

'I was refused HRT.' — Tina

Take Tina's story. Her periods were erratic for about two years up until a year ago, when she describes developing a raft of symptoms like 'flicking on a switch'.

Rapid hair loss, full-on body aches, memory loss/brain fog, trouble sleeping, constant headaches, night sweats, extreme stomach ache, constant periods and tiredness.

I spoke to my GP who felt I was too young to be going through the menopause at forty-nine years old. Finally, I rang the GP again – by that time I'd lost half of my hair – and I demanded to see them. They confirmed I was going through the menopause, but I refused HRT due to the risks of breast cancer.

Watching Davina's documentary changed my mind. When I rang the doctor and asked to be put on HRT they initially declined (it was a different doctor this time). I refused to accept this, complained, and they changed their mind and prescribed it to me.

Two weeks after applying the patch, Tina says most of her symptoms 'vanished' and she realised how much she had been suffering.

Tina, thanks so much for sharing your story. I too realised after I started taking HRT that I had been suffering in many more ways than I had been aware of, because it was only when I started feeling better that I could see how bad I'd been feeling. So thank you very much for sharing that, I know women will identify with your story.

There is so much fear surrounding something that has the power to literally transform lives.

Where do these myths come from? And what are the real facts? We need them NOW.

This chapter is all about setting the record straight. We'll be looking at:

→ The Women's Health Initiative (WHI): how one study set back women's health care for decades.

→ What science says about HRT today.

→ Dr Naomi's HRT myth-busters, including: can I take HRT if I've had breast cancer? What about if there is a family history of breast cancer? I've had DVT – can I take HRT?

→ What to do if your doctor won't prescribe HRT.

WHI: HOW ONE STUDY SET BACK WOMEN'S HEALTH CARE FOR DECADES

Remember that stat at the start of the last chapter: only 10 per cent of women who would benefit from HRT in the UK actually take it.[1] Flip this on its head for a moment. That's nearly nine out of every ten women who could have it, but DON'T.

The picture isn't much better in other parts of the world, either. One study found about 13 per cent of post-menopausal women in Australia take HRT, for example.[2]

It's outrageous that more women don't have access to it if they want to take it. But why not? This can be through choice, but also lack of knowledge and lack of support. Now the name WHI might not be familiar, but you'll undoubtedly have seen the headlines about it.

The WHI was a large clinical trial that started in the USA in 1993. The aim of the trial was to look at the health effects on thousands of women taking oestrogen-only or combined HRT.

But in 2002, the combined HRT arm of the study was suddenly halted amid findings of an increased risk of breast cancer, heart disease, stroke and blood clots among the 16,000 women taking combined HRT in the trial.

The findings were released and caused a media storm, making front-page news around the world. It alleged that breast cancer increased by 26 per cent when women took combined HRT, while the risk of heart disease, stroke and blood clots also increased.[3]

Unsurprisingly, the impact of these findings and how they were reported in the media was absolutely devastating.

Even though I was nowhere near my perimenopause and menopause years at the time, I can distinctly recall just how frightening those headlines were. Everyone was talking about it. I remember thinking to myself 'God, HRT causes breast cancer.'

---

[1] G.P Cumming, et al. (2015) 'The need to do better – Are we still letting our patients down and at what cost?', Post Reproductive Health, 21 (2), pp. 56–62. Doi.org/10.1177/2053369115586122

[2] L.S. Velentzis, E. Banks, F. Sitas, U. Salagame, E.H. Tan, K. Canfell (2016), 'Use of menopausal hormone therapy and bioidentical hormone therapy in Australian women 50 to 69 years of age: results from a national, cross-sectional study, PLoS One, doi.org/10.1371/journal.pone.0146494

[3] Women's Health Initiative (2019), 'Hormone therapy trials', www.whi.org/about/SitePages/HT.aspx

And I wasn't the only one who thought that. The coverage caused mass panic and, pretty much overnight, women stopped taking HRT and doctors stopped prescribing it. Between 2003 and 2007 in the UK alone, the numbers of women on HRT plummeted from two million to one million.[3]

The labels that 'HRT causes breast cancer', that 'HRT is unsafe' stuck, right up to the present day.

WHAT WAS WRONG WITH THE STUDY?

But when we look more closely at the study, there were flaws in its design:[4]

1. It only looked at one dose and type of combined and at one dose and type of oestrogen-only HRT. In addition, the oestrogen was an older, oral type and the progestogen was also an older type. As we know from Dr Naomi's HRT masterclass in the last chapter, HRT is not a one-size-fits-all treatment. There are literally dozens of different combinations and dosages that are tailored to you and your health.

2. The mean age of women participating in the trial was sixty-three years – more than a decade older than fifty-one, the average age of menopause. In fact, the oldest women involved in the trial were aged seventy-nine. This means that, due to their age, the women already had an increased risk of breast cancer and cardiovascular events.

3. Because the trial was stopped early, the preliminary findings were incorrectly applied to all age groups, including lower-risk women in their late forties and fifties.

4. The majority of the women in the study were overweight. Being overweight increases the risk of heart disease, breast cancer and other cancers.

5. There was a substantial number of drop-outs from the study.

WHAT WE CAN LEARN FROM THE WHI

The WHI study was huge and it does contain a lot of useful information. Re-analysis of the data gives us a more accurate picture. In the fifty- to fifty-nine-year age group, there was no increased risk of death from heart disease or breast cancer.

However, the controversy around the initial report is still felt to this day.

[4] Women's Health Concern (2020). 'HRT: the history' www.womens-health-concern.org/help-and-advice/factsheets/hrt-the-history/

SO, WHAT DO WE KNOW ABOUT THE REAL RISK OF HRT AND BREAST CANCER TODAY?

The latest study confirms what we already thought was the case that oestrogen-only HRT does not increase the risk of breast cancer. Oestrogen plus micronised (body-identical) progesterone is also not associated with an increased risk of breast cancer. Oestrogen with synthetic progesterone is associated with a small increased risk of breast cancer.[5]

Twenty-three out of 1,000 women aged between fifty and fifty-nine will develop breast cancer over the next five years. In comparison, twenty-seven out of 1,000 women aged fifty and fifty-nine will develop breast cancer if they use combined HRT with a synthetic progesterone. By comparison, twenty-eight women out of 1,000 in the same age group will develop breast cancer if they drink two or more units of alcohol a day. And the most telling statistic, forty-seven women out of 1,000 aged fifty and fifty-nine will develop breast cancer if they are overweight or obese.[6]

If you exercise for two and a half hours a week you can reduce your risk of breast cancer by the same degree as combined HRT with synthetic progesterone increases it.[5]

ARE THERE ANY OTHER RISKS WITH HRT THAT I NEED TO KNOW ABOUT?

There is a slightly increased risk of developing a blood clot if you take **oral** oestrogen. There is **no** increased risk of blood clots from using oestrogen through the skin. The leaflets inside the packets of HRT are inaccurate as they advise that transdermal HRT increases this risk, but that is not the case.

Studies show that transdermal HRT (through the skin) does not significantly increase the risk of cardiovascular disease, including heart disease and strokes, if you start taking it before sixty years of age.[7]

NOTE: Although every attempt has been made to ensure the advice on the right is accurate, it should not be used to substitute the input and advice from your own doctor.

---

[5] Women's Health Concern (2020). 'HRT: the history' www.womens-health-concern.org/help-and-advice/factsheets/hrt-the-history/

[6] Women's Health Concern (2019), 'Breast cancer risk factors', www.womens-health-concern.org/help-and-advice/factsheets/breast-cancer-risk-factors/

[7] NICE (2015), 'Menopause: diagnosis and management', www.nice.org.uk/guidance/ng23

Who CAN have transdermal HRT?

STILL HAVING PERIODS

NOT HAVING PERIODS

UNDER FORTY-FIVE

OVER FIFTY-FIVE

OVERWEIGHT

HIGH BLOOD PRESSURE

HISTORY OF CLOTS

FAMILY HISTORY OF BREAST CANCER
(MOST OF THE TIME)

HISTORY OF MOST CANCERS

OCCASIONALLY EVEN WITH BREAST CANCER

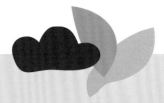

DR NAOMI:
HRT MYTH-BUSTERS

If you are still concerned about HRT and its bad press, here's Dr Naomi to answer all those burning questions and dispel the most common myths.

DOESN'T HRT JUST DELAY THE INEVITABLE?

Nope. HRT replaces hormones that are fluctuating and falling, stopping the symptoms. If you choose to come off HRT for whatever reason, you can do so slowly to reduce symptoms or prevent them returning.

CAN I TAKE HRT IF I HAVE MIGRAINES?

Yes, but I'd exercise some caution with the dose and delivery method.

Migraines can worsen during perimenopause and menopause because of the hormone fluctuations, so it's a good idea to start gently on a lower dose to see what happens with those migraines and adjust accordingly. Also, it's better to have a continuous regime rather than a cyclical one – in this instance a Mirena coil can be preferable.

If you suffer from a migraine with aura (the type where you get a warning sign that a migraine is on its way, such as visual symptoms) you do have a slightly higher baseline risk of developing a clot, so it's better to use a transdermal form of oestrogen.

Women who have migraine with aura also shouldn't take the contraceptive pill, but this is because the pill uses a different oestrogen usually at a higher dose.

I HAVE HIGH BLOOD PRESSURE. CAN I TAKE HRT?

The short answer is yes, but it depends. High blood pressure is not a reason to refuse HRT outright. HRT can be cardio-protective – it can protect the heart and vessels from furring up, and it helps keep blood vessels soft and flexible. If you are perimenopausal or not far into menopause it can actually help your blood pressure, but if you are ten years post-menopause or in your late sixties or seventies it may not be suitable. The important thing to remember is that every situation is different, so it depends on your age and cardiovascular risk.

Your doctor should be treating you as a whole, looking to treat your high blood pressure and your menopause symptoms. If your blood pressure is very high, then your doctor should be investigating the cause and how to bring it down, but in many cases I would start HRT simultaneously with the treatment for blood pressure.

I HAVE A HISTORY OF CLOTS. DOES THAT MEAN HRT IS COMPLETELY OFF LIMITS?

It's a myth that women with a history of clots are unable to take any HRT.

Yes, oral oestrogen slightly increases the risk of clots, so if you have a history of clots, you definitely shouldn't take oral oestrogen. But transdermal oestrogen, and topical oestrogen for vaginal dryness, do not carry the same risk.

The same goes for micronised, body-identical progestogen. It does not carry an increased risk of clot and is safe.

When a patient has a history of clots, I always delve much more deeply into the history of that clot. Was it triggered by something like a long-haul flight, or do they have a clotting disorder?

The general rule of thumb is that if you aren't having to take anti-coagulants, then you can use transdermal oestrogen and micronised progestogen.

We often liaise with haematology over cases such as this. Sometimes we identify women who haven't been anticoagulated who should have been and vice versa but as long as they are on the correct medication for their clotting disorder, adding transdermal HRT should not make them more likely to suffer clots.

WHAT ABOUT IF I SMOKE?

Your doctor should be prescribing transdermal HRT – patches, gels, sprays – as this does not increase the risk of clots.

You could use this as an ideal time to stop. Not only is it terrible all round for your health, but smoking can also increase hot flushes and make them last longer.[8]

---

[8] L. Gallicchio, et al. (2006), 'Cigarette smoking, estrogen levels, and hot flashes in midlife women', Maturitas, 53 (2) pp.133-43, doi.org/10.1016/j.maturitas.2005.03.007

OR I LIKE A GLASS OF WINE...?

Generally speaking, perimenopause and menopause symptoms and alcohol don't tend to mix. Alcohol can make symptoms like hot flushes worse, it can interrupt your sleep and make you feel more anxious than you were already, and a hangover can leave you craving sugar. While you can still drink alcohol while taking HRT, now might be the perfect time to assess if you really are drinking in moderation.

HRT AND A FAMILY OR PERSONAL HISTORY OF CANCER

Women with cancer, especially with a history of breast and gynaecological cancer, can often feel overlooked when it comes to menopause care.

It's very common for women with any personal or family history of cancer to be told they can't have HRT under any circumstances. However, this may not always be the case, and it means some women who have severe symptoms and who could benefit from HRT are left to struggle on.

If you have a history of cancer, I'd recommend that you see someone with specialist knowledge to discuss your options. It is important that you have a discussion about your own personal circumstances and weigh up the risks and benefits. It is about teasing out what is the right way forward in every single case.

It is also worth remembering that if HRT is not suitable, there are alternatives, which are covered in Chapter 11, that can help bring relief from symptoms like hot flushes, vaginal and urinary symptoms, as well as lifestyle adjustments.

I'VE HAD BREAST CANCER. CAN I TAKE HRT?

Not all breast cancers are the same. Some cancers are hormone-receptor positive, which means tumours may grow under the influence of hormones. About seventy-five per cent of all breast cancers have receptors for oestrogen and are called oestrogen-receptor positive or ER positive (ER+) breast cancer.[9] Officially, HRT is contraindicated (not advised as a course of treatment) for any woman with a history of breast cancer. However, sometimes if a woman

---

[9] Cancer Research UK (2020), 'Tests on Your Breast Cancer Cells', https://www.cancerresearchuk.org/about-cancer/breast-cancer/getting-diagnosed/tests-diagnose/hormone-receptor-testing-breast-cancer

had breast cancer a very long time ago, or it was very localised, it might be possible to take HRT under the guidance of a specialist. What is key here is looking at a patient's individual history and weighing up the pros and cons of HRT.

If your cancer was not hormone-dependent, then it may be relatively safe to give HRT under the guidance of a specialist.

WHAT ABOUT A FAMILY HISTORY OF BREAST CANCER?

Women with a family history of breast cancer are often told they can't take HRT, which in fact is often not the case. If you have a strong family history of breast cancer (for example, your mum or sister was diagnosed with breast cancer before the age of forty) you are more likely to develop breast cancer, but it is not thought that HRT will increase your risk further. Again, I would advise speaking to a specialist before deciding on whether to take HRT. In addition, if you are worried about your family history of breast cancer, you can also ask your GP for a referral to a

specialist family history clinic or a regional genetics centre which could help you to find out more.

CERVICAL, VULVA AND VAGINA CANCER

If you have had cervical, vulva or vagina cancer it is normally safe to use HRT. There are some exceptions, but of course speak to your specialist.

ENDOMETRIAL CANCER

For women with early-stage endometrial cancer (cancer of the lining of the womb), stages 1 and 2, one study suggests there is no increase in risk of recurrence from HRT.[10] However, at the moment there is not enough clear data for more advanced endometrial cancer, so specialists are cautious in prescribing HRT.

OVARIAN CANCER

Ovarian cancer is more complicated as it will depend on the type of cancer, because some are hormone-receptor positive. You should definitely discuss your individual benefits and risks with a specialist.

[10] K.A Edey, et al. (2018), 'Hormone replacement therapy for women previously treated for endometrial cancer', The Cochrane Database of Systematic Reviews, 5 (5), doi.org/10.1002/14651858.CD008830.pub3

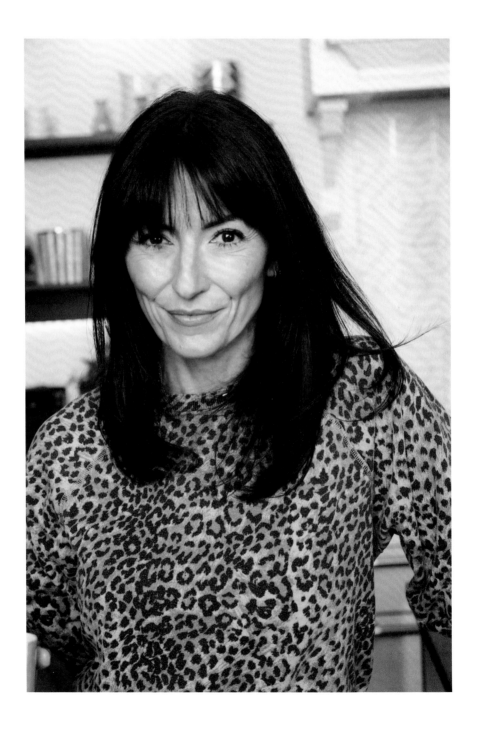

WANT TO TALK HRT? MY GUIDE TO DISCUSSING IT WITH YOUR DOCTOR

GPs are doctors who specialize in general medicine. They are dedicated and knowledgeable professionals who do such an important job and want to do the best by their patients. However, I do hear from my own patients, women on social media and, of course, those of you who have generously shared your experiences for this book, that it is not always easy to access HRT through your local surgery.

There are various reasons for this. First is the lack of training: a 2021 survey of thirty-three UK medical schools found forty-one per cent did not have mandatory menopause education on the curriculum.[11] Menopause training for both GPs and gynaecologists alike is seriously lacking.

Then there is the lack of time. GPs face seeing dozens of patients every day and have only minutes to make an assessment.

The WHI study still casts a shadow to this day, causing confusion on whether HRT is the right choice for patients. The headlines around the breast cancer risk in particular have stuck, and a GP will not want to prescribe something they believe will harm their patient, even if the evidence now suggests this really isn't the case.

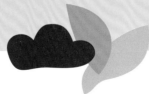

'I'm hopeful the person I used to be will come back.' — Michelle

Michelle experienced a blood clot after giving birth to her son, and from that day on, she was told HRT was not going to be an option. But when menopause hit, she persevered to get help so she could safely manage her symptoms.

Back in 2000 I gave birth to my son and a few days later I was diagnosed with a blood clot. I was on anticoagulants for about six months, and I recovered well. At the time, I was told HRT would be off the table for me in the future because of the blood clot. I absorbed this snippet of info then forgot about it.

In 2017, I started to feel very different – and not in a good way. I visited my GP and when I asked about whether HRT would be an option, I was very clearly told the risk to me was far too great – why would I risk it? 'Many people have menopause and deal with it themselves,' she said. I should weigh up the small inconvenience of hot flushes and other symptoms compared to the high risk that HRT would have on me. I was told menopause won't last forever!

I felt like I was asking for the world, and feeling rather pathetic, I left thinking I must just accept this and get on with it, like other women do. I cut out caffeine, cut down on alcohol to once a week, exercised more, took supplements, and

did anything and everything I could. I had terrible brain fog and felt like a woman possessed. Barely functioning on little sleep, I couldn't bear my husband's voice, let alone being intimate, so I kept my distance. He didn't understand. I was the butt of jokes for being forgetful and because of my hot flushes. This made me depressed, desperate and hopeless.

In 2019 I went back to my surgery and I saw an old favourite GP by chance. I told him I couldn't cope and practically broke down. He wrote to my specialist at the hospital who confirmed HRT patches were an option if I needed it. I was still sceptical because of the risks. I sat on it for a while longer to see how I got on. After watching the documentary, I thought, why am I worried? The specialist said I can have HRT, and listening to the science and statistics I decided to contact my GP and take him up on the offer. I'm now a few months in and on a very low dose so the jury is out if this will be enough, but I feel better already. My fog is starting to clear, sleep is also improving, and I am hopeful the person I used to be will soon make a comeback. Look out, husband!

Thank you, Michelle, for your story. It's very important to talk about blood clots and people that suffer with blood clots, so thank you so much for sharing that.

'I'm a GP and I'm still struggling to get HRT prescribed on the NHS.' — Paula

It tells you something about the state of affairs if Paula – a doctor who got in touch – struggled to get HRT for herself. Here's her story:

I qualified as a doctor in 2005 and had deep vein thrombosis in about 2009. I've always had heavy, painful periods and I noticed a change in them about five years ago. I went to my GP practice and asked whether the changes were due to oestrogen and was dismissed at least twice, including by a women's health expert at the practice.

In the end I had to access HRT privately and I'm still struggling to get it prescribed on the NHS. If as a doctor I can't get it then I worry about other women.

One thing I am glad for is that as a GP I've been able to advise friends how to access HRT and as a result their doctors have prescribed it for them, and they have benefited.

Paula, thanks so much for telling your story. It's so interesting to hear it from a GP's point of view as well.

'I put up with hot flushes and night sweats for years.' — Lesley

Lesley shared her story about a pretty shocking experience with her doctor. The solution? She had to wait until he was on holiday before she could get the prescription she needed.

I started to have hot flushes at fifty, and all other symptoms associated with menopause. It was the night sweats that finally forced me to see my doctor. He drew me a picture of my head with some little dots and said, 'there's your problem', like I was imagining it!

I put up with hot flushes and night sweats for five years, trying every natural cure under the sun, none of which helped. I went back and asked the receptionist if I could see another doctor. I finally managed to see another doctor when mine was on holiday, and she prescribed HRT.

Your story infuriates me, Lesley. I can't believe you struggled on for five years. I am glad that you finally got prescribed HRT and are now able to sleep, but this still never really needs to happen.

Even if it isn't in your nature, this is the point where you need to push.

Never be afraid to ask your doctor why. What are they basing the decision on? Is it in line with NICE guidelines? Are they considering your circumstances, your symptoms and your wishes? Could they discuss their decision with a colleague?

If you are unhappy, you can absolutely ask for a second opinion. This could be simply asking to see a different doctor, or pushing for a referral to an NHS menopause clinic. Alternatively, you can change practice or see a private menopause specialist.

If you are visiting the GP for the first time about your symptoms, and especially if you are wanting to try HRT, here are some tips on making the situation work for you:

→ Make a list of your symptoms, with the most pressing ones at the top.

→ Ask for a recommendation when booking your appointment. The receptionist may be able to direct you to who they would recommend you see to discuss perimenopause or menopause.

→ GP registrars, who are doctors training to be GPs, are a good place to start as they are normally up to date with the latest training and keen to learn.

→ Book a double appointment (if you can, whether face-to-face or by telephone) – appointments can fly by, so give yourself a bit of breathing space.

→ Print off a copy of the NICE menopause guidelines (www.nice. org.uk/guidance/ng23, or available at my website www.menopausecare. co.uk). These were developed in 2015 for healthcare professionals around menopause, covering symptoms, diagnosis and treatment.

They recommend HRT as the first-line treatment for menopausal symptoms.

→ The appointment can be quite emotionally draining, so take a friend or relative with you who can support you, ask questions and take notes.

→ If anxiety or depression are part of your symptoms, explain that these are symptoms you have never experienced before. Make a list of your symptoms.

→ If you are offered bloods, show the NICE guidelines.

→ Oestrogen: ideally, do some research beforehand and make a decision about what kind of oestrogen product you want to try.

→ Progesterone: think about which progesterone product you want to use. Mirena coil? Body-identical progesterone?

→ If you are experiencing urinary or vaginal symptoms, remember you can use topical oestrogens if your systemic oestrogen doesn't seem to be helping, or your symptoms are more severe.

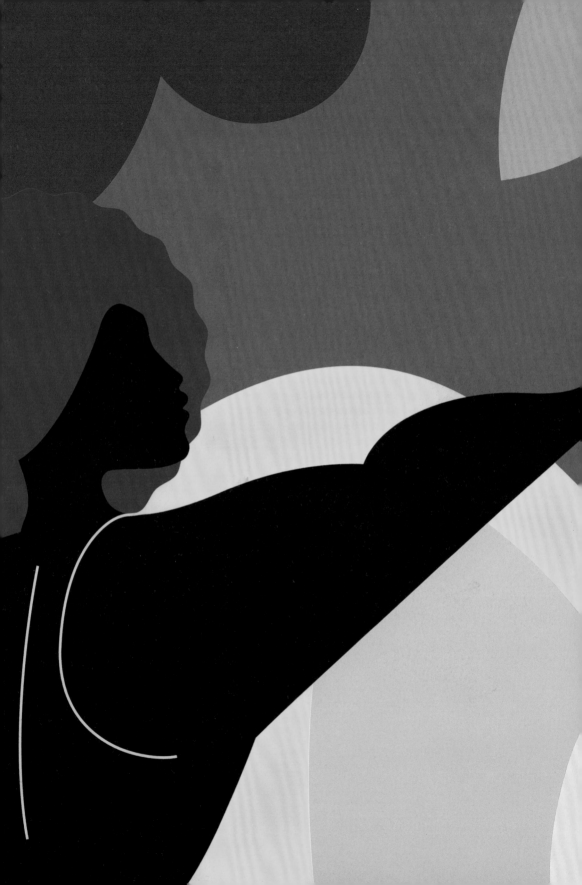

CHAPTER 7

DOCTOR, DOCTOR ... I'M NOT DEPRESSED, I'M MENOPAUSAL

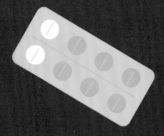

1 in 4 women have been prescribed antidepressants for menopause symptoms.[1]

During my evenings on Twitter, talking to and learning from peri-, post- and menopausal women, the one issue I hear about night after night after night is depression.

Looking back on my own journey, if I'm honest I was probably a bit down, too, only I didn't see it as that at the time. I didn't really have an answer or a reason for it. I just thought I was a bit 'down' or a bit off.

The French call it *malaise*, like a sadness that creeps in very, very slowly and suddenly it's there sitting on your shoulder. The sad thing is that so many women will just accept these feelings, thinking 'Oh, it's my age' and resign themselves to it.

It's a bit like the aches and pains we put down to getting older, where you think 'Well, I suppose I should get used to it as I am getting on a bit.'

Sorry, but no. Bollocks to that. Being depressed is *not* something you have to put up with on account of your age.

We have to talk about these feelings, and we have to support women experiencing them and give them the right help. Because if we don't, lives are literally at risk.

Do you know that women between the ages of forty-five and fifty-four have the highest suicide rate of any female age group?[2] For every 100,000 women in that age group, seven will take their own life. That's more than double the suicide rate of those aged fifteen to nineteen.[2] In sixty-five to sixty-nine-year-olds it falls to 3.7 per 100,000 women.[2]

These are really frightening stats.

I've heard from teenagers who have lost their mums to suicide because they couldn't cope any more. It's absolutely heartbreaking.

But the one thing I've learned from talking to women and doctors (there are lots of doctors and other specialists also spending their evenings trying to help menopausal women online) is this: if low mood and depression is hormonal, then HRT is the first-line treatment.[3]

But even so, when listening to you all, antidepressants continue to be given to women with menopause-related depression, anxiety and mood changes.

A survey of 5,000 perimenopausal and menopausal women as recently as 2021 found that one in four were given antidepressants. However, the NICE menopause guidelines are very clear

[1] Newson Health and Education (2021), 'Delayed diagnosis and treatment of menopause is wasting NHS appointments and resources', www.balance-menopause.com/news/delayed-diagnosis-and-treatment-of-menopause-is-wasting-nhs-appointments-and-resources/

[2] Office for National Statistics (2021), Suicides in England and Wales: 2020 registrations', www.ons.gov.uk/peoplepopulationandcommunity/birthsdeathsandmarriages/deaths/bulletins/suicidesintheunitedkingdom/2020registrations

[3] NICE (2015), 'Menopause: diagnosis and management', www.nice.org.uk/guidance/ng23

that menopause symptoms should be treated first with HRT and not antidepressants.

The danger is that if a hormonal woman is treated with antidepressants and they don't work, it can leave her feeling even more scared and confused. Then they get prescribed something stronger, or different, and perhaps it still doesn't work. They think, if the tablets aren't working, what is wrong with me?

If, like me, you were born in the 1960s (or earlier), you'll probably recall that in the sixties there was an absolute pandemic of housewives being prescribed Valium for anxiety, insomnia or to help with the stresses of modern life. Between the late sixties and the early eighties, Valium was the most prescribed drug in the USA.[4] 'Mother's little helper', they called it.

But it *must* have been menopause. That was perimenopausal and menopausal women all struggling and seeking help, but instead they were handed a pill so they could disappear from life in a sort of plush velvet blanket.

Constantly over the decades we use prescription drugs to placate without stopping to look at the root cause.

Every single night without fail I have three or four women telling me how they've gone to the doctor and been prescribed antidepressants, even though they are adamant they aren't depressed. They *know* they aren't clinically depressed. So why do they keep being given antidepressants?

· · · · · · ·

'Anxiety was my worst symptom.' — Margaret

Mental health was a common thread through your stories. Margaret was forty-two when her menopause started, and anxiety was her first symptom. She describes feeling constantly worried, even though she says she had nothing to worry about:

I had all the symptoms; physical and mental, but the anxiety was by far the worst. I went to several doctors and explained everything but nobody could help me. My marriage broke down, I had to give up work and I basically lost the will to live.

---

[4] American Addiction Centers Drugabuse.com (2021), 'Valium history and statistics', www.drugabuse.com/benzodiazepines/valium/history-and-statistics

I started HRT three months ago and my mental health has vastly improved.

Often depression and anxiety, as I've said earlier in the book, are huge signs of perimenopause – so, Margaret, thanks very much for your story and we're so glad to hear that you're feeling better.

'My mood has been on the floor.' — Gillian

Gillian went into surgical menopause aged thirty-nine after having an ovary removed due to a dermoid cyst. She says she wasn't given enough information about what it would mean to go into menopause and was left to figure it out alone.

My mood has been on the floor a lot of the time, and when I asked my GP for help and to review my HRT she decided to prescribe me Prozac after a ten-minute phone consultation. I feel I am on my own, working it out by myself with very little support.

Thank you so much for your story, Gillian. I am hoping, seriously, that there are women who will read this book before they go into surgical menopause, because it is really important to know all the facts about what you're going to need after your surgical menopause, and to ask your surgeon or specialist to recommend you or refer you to a menopause clinic or specialist after your op. Thank you so much.

'Why are we not taught about this, when we will all experience it in our lives?' — Gilly

When Gilly became overwhelmed by everyday tasks like renewing her car insurance, found it increasingly harder to retain information and started wondering if some hip pain might be pointing to perimenopause, she contacted her doctor.

I first spoke to a locum GP in September 2020 in a phone consultation (Covid-19 meant no face-to-face appointments). She didn't listen.

By then I also had anxiety every evening. My heart felt like it was beating out of my chest. I had initially thought this might be pandemic-related as I am such a social person and work in a theatre, and the pandemic had really affected me.

The GP offered me antidepressants and told me to stop drinking coffee. This consultation made me feel very angry. I did cut out coffee and felt no different.

I then read up on menopause and asked for another phone consultation with a different GP. The doctor was very nice but didn't want to prescribe me HRT at all, and cited breast cancer risks.

He suggested I go and think about it, and that if I did want an HRT trial I could ask for one and he would prescribe it as I'd done my research.

So I waited a bit longer and it was the week before Davina's TV programme aired and she'd done an Instagram live. I was so fired up and sent a tweet to Davina about HRT, and she replied and told me to go for it.

The very next day, I called the surgery and asked to speak to the same GP. I asked specifically for body-identical HRT and I got my prescription that day.

It took just a few days to begin to feel the benefits. My brain came back to life, I felt like 'me', my spark was back, my joint pain went in just a week and over a two-month period almost all the heart palpitations went.

I have just signed up to volunteer with the Menopause Charity as I feel so strongly that women get informed. Why are we not taught about this, when we will all experience it in our lives?

Gilly, thank you so much for your story. Yes, the anxiety manifests itself in such strange ways, doesn't it? Quite a few people have said that they weren't anxious at all about things like driving at night, or large crowds of people, or walking home from the corner shop at dusk, and all of a sudden they got this anxiety. They put it down to ageing – this is how people feel when they get older. But actually it's not, it's the hormones. I'm so pleased that you watched the Instagram Live and it helped in some way, and fantastic for signing up to the Menopause Charity to help out there. Well done!

'The kids told their teachers that "mummy was always crying".' — Dora

For Dora, lockdown and a subsequent car accident brought her to breaking point.

Anxiety has hit hard, physically waking me up in the night, causing me to feel panicked and shaking. Every night, I found myself pacing the house, adrenaline rushing through my body, knowing I soon had to get up and face the school run, housework and job hunting. I completely lost my confidence, my mind, my sanity.

Somehow, I managed to wing a new sales job at the start of 2021, but then another lockdown hit and the schools closed during my first week.

I struggled SO much: crying more than I have ever done before, forgetting words and meetings. The kids told their teachers that 'mummy was always crying', so the school got in touch to offer us counselling.

The brain fog hit me hard, and work were awful about it. I was head of sales and could hardly cope with a job I'd been doing for twenty years. I had no support, and every mistake I made was broadcast to senior staff. I worked until late at night. I was exhausted. I was constantly tired

and ended up having a car accident and rolling the car with the kids inside.

My employers insisted I make back the time I had to take off work after the accident. In the end, I left. They insinuated I couldn't cope. My husband thought it was all in my head and that I'm too young for menopause: but I'm forty-five, and my mum went through menopause at forty-two.

Finally, after a cervical cancer scare, being refused HRT and watching Davina's documentary, I insisted on a referral to a specialist menopause clinic.

I have to say that in writing this book and reading all your stories, I have sobbed, literally, sitting here. And Dora, I am horrified by what you have been through. Going through it alone, unsupported, too. I really hope – and I'd love to hear back from you, Dora – that the specialist menopause clinic helped you. But please stay in touch.

'I'm just a normal, middle-aged woman who wants to talk about menopause and mental health.' — Sally-Anne

Sally-Anne suffered from mental health issues in her teens and was hospitalised with postpartum psychosis after the birth of her first child.

For the next twenty years, she says she kept relatively well, aside from insomnia in her late thirties, and PMS, which was alleviated by a Mirena coil.

About two years ago Sally-Anne started to have hot flushes but thought she was coping. She went on HRT, which helped her sleep, but still wasn't perfect.

I'm now menopausal. Two years ago I was admitted to a psychiatric hospital for the first time since 2001. I have been medicated, therapised and am still on HRT. I'm trying to get the balance of HRT right.

I recovered and was doing pretty well but then ended up back in hospital. I'm at my wits' end with this!

I'm British but am currently living in Ireland, where I am receiving good care but struggling to convince the psychiatrists of what seems to me to

be a pretty bloody obvious link between times of great hormonal flux and extreme mental health problems.

I want to stress to women just how extreme the effects of hormone shift can be on your mental health. I'm not a 'I was running the United Nations but then my brain turned to mush'-type woman, I'm just a normal, middle-aged woman who turned fifty last week who wants to talk about menopause and mental health.

Sally-Anne, thanks so much for your story. As a patient who is suffering so greatly with your mental health and with your other issues, it seems so obvious to you, and to me reading this, that it would be worth exploring the effect of hormones on your mental health. I love that last line: *I'm just a normal, middle-aged woman who turned fifty last week who wants to talk about menopause and mental health.* That's all of us, and we're all right behind you.

As well as hormones, there are so many different aspects that can feed into feelings of anxiety and depression during menopause. First there's the sleep deprivation. Then there's anxiety over the unknown, that overwhelming feeling that something is out of kilter in your body, but you can't quite put your finger on exactly what it is.

Memory lapses and brain fogginess also lead to anxiety. That brain fog gives you a niggling feeling that something hasn't been done, that you've forgotten to do something really important, or you just aren't 'with it'.

Now I'm no psychologist, and I'm not a scientist either, but I think that part of my low mood stemmed from the feeling that menopause was the end of a chapter in my life; the end of something. Grieving, in a way.

When I realised I was menopausal, I grieved for the fact I wasn't able to have any more children. It wasn't that I *wanted* any more children – in fact, I knew I didn't. Yet menopause still represented a door closing on that part of my life and there was a period of time when I had to come to terms with that.

The end of that chapter isn't just about biology, it says something about your femininity, how you are as a person. In menopause you have to reassess how you see yourself as a woman. I know not every woman will feel like this, but from when I was about seventeen years old, I just felt I was meant to make babies. And for a time, it felt like my purpose in life had just vanished, too.

This chapter is about lifting the lid on mental health during perimenopause and menopause. The treatments that will help, the ones that won't – how to get the treatment you need and what to do if you are faced with resistance.

Remember, when you are informed, you are empowered to make the right choices for you.

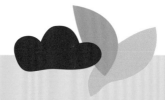

DR NAOMI: WHY ANTIDEPRESSANTS AREN'T USUALLY THE ANSWER FOR MENOPAUSE-RELATED MOOD PROBLEMS

Antidepressants are widely used to treat depression because they can be very effective – but this is a different diagnosis to hormonally-induced low mood.

While it is true that the range of mood changes in perimenopause and menopause – anxiety, depression, anger, irritability, tearfulness – can overlap with depression, the key difference is that menopause symptoms are linked to hormones.

Falling oestrogen levels directly impact the production of brain chemicals that help to regulate mood.

Antidepressants definitely have their role, but in menopause HRT has consistently proven to be the most effective way of treating mood disorders in women who are able to take it.

SO WHY DO ANTIDEPRESSANTS KEEP BEING OFFERED TO MENOPAUSAL WOMEN?

This is a very real problem, and it is a combination of a lack of in-depth menopause training for healthcare professionals, and time. GPs seeing patients with mental-health-type symptoms may routinely prescribe antidepressants and may not necessarily link the symptoms to menopause. GPs have very little time to spend with a patient to unpick what is potentially a very complex network of symptoms, and if menopause does not spring to mind, it may not occur to them.

HOW TO GET THE RIGHT TREATMENT FIRST TIME

As we know, doctor appointments are short, so you want to be clear straight away about your symptoms and that you believe them to be menopause-related, to avoid wasting valuable time in getting a diagnosis.

→ Mention the perimenopause or menopause word so it is at the forefront of the conversation.

→ Be very clear about the symptoms you are experiencing, so your doctor can build up as detailed a picture as possible. If the symptoms come and go, then make a point of saying this.

→ If you feel low or anxious but you don't think you have depression, make that clear.

→ State what treatment approaches you want to try, such as HRT.

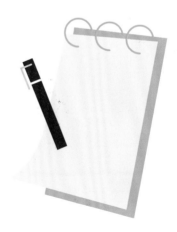

Offered antidepressants? FIVE key questions to ask your doctor:

WHY are these being prescribed?

AM I depressed?

HOW are these going to help me?

COULD I have HRT instead?

And if you aren't happy with the answers you are getting:

CAN I see someone else?

COPING STRATEGIES

Mood problems should start to improve within four days to three months of starting HRT. Testosterone can take up to four months to work.

But there are some other strategies you can try – some of them today, *right now* – to help you through.

COGNITIVE BEHAVIOURAL THERAPY (CBT)

CBT is a type of talking therapy that helps you identify and change unhelpful thought patterns. It's used for a range of mental health conditions, but it's a therapy recommended in the NICE menopause guidelines for menopause-related mood changes and can also help with hot flushes.

You can ask to be referred to your local service by your GP, or you might want to see someone privately. Courses might be online, as group therapy or one-to-one.

I have heard amazing things about CBT. I haven't personally done it but I hear that it really works wonders, especially for women who can't take HRT for medical reasons. So CBT should be top of your list if you are waiting for the HRT to work, or if you can't take it.

MINDFULNESS

Mindfulness is all about training your mind to block out all the noise from the world around you and focus on the present moment.

I love mindfulness and I've practised it on and off for about nine or ten years now, but it really came into its own during that first Covid lockdown in 2020. The schools were closed, work was on hold, I'd worry that even going to the supermarket was unsafe and I'd lie there at night feeling anxious about the state of the world or wake up early with a knot in my stomach. I couldn't face watching TV or listening to music, which was a weird thing for me because I usually love doing both of those things.

I had to do things for my sanity's sake, so I started doing mindfulness again. I downloaded the Headspace app (www.headspace.com) and did guided meditations for about ten minutes every day.

It was really, really amazing, like putting fuel back in the tank. And because I was being kinder to myself, I felt more present, and I was a better mum and friend as a result.

Don't just take my word for it; studies have shown that mindfulness can help depression, anxiety, insomnia and even hot flushes during menopause.[5]

GET MOVING

Ok, it's no surprise that I put this very high on the list of things that are going to help you.

Exercise is amazing for your mental health. It helps you sleep, manages stress, calms down a racing mind, gives you a massive sense of accomplishment and something to focus on … the list goes on and on.

I call exercise my workout for my body **and** my mind. Even if you get out for twenty minutes to half an hour, to walk the dog, or yourself, or anyone – just feel some fresh air on your face and get out, come rain or shine. Sometimes my favourite dog walks are the ones in the rain.

To just feel the fresh air on your face and that gust of wind whooshing through your hair – being connected to nature can be so healing. Even if you live in a city, you can connect to nature there: look up at the sky, feel the sun, look at the birds, hear the sounds, go watch the sunrise … connect.

Exercise also releases endorphins, those feel-good chemicals that promote a feeling of physical and mental wellbeing. Chapter 12 has got some really brilliant menopause-friendly exercises just to get you started.

'Going on walks during lockdown saved me.' — Paula

If you're unconvinced about the benefits of walking for your mental health, please read Paula's story.

When she was forty-nine, in addition to irregular periods, she started to have hot flushes. She was feeling low, suffering from anxiety, low self-esteem, paranoia and wasn't sleeping.

I went to my GP as I thought my thyroid levels weren't right, but when the blood tests to check my thyroid levels came back normal, I was referred for CBT.

I stopped running due to sore knees and sciatica. I began to feel out of control. I was short-tempered and was hell to live with. At work, I had totally lost

---

[5] C. Wong et al. (2018), 'Mindfulness-Based Stress Reduction (MBSR) or psychoeducation for the reduction of menopausal symptoms: a randomized, controlled clinical trial', Scientific Reports, 8(1), doi.org/10.1038/s41598-018-24945-4

my confidence and I couldn't retain anything. My dad has Alzheimer's and was in a home.

I just wasn't coping, and in February 2020 I had a total meltdown – I completely lost it. I walked out the house, got in my car and drove like a lunatic, crying hysterically, hyperventilating, trying to work out how I could run away.

Then Covid and lockdown happened and ironically the first lockdown saved me. I started going on long walks, which was great for my mental health.

Thank you, Paula, for your story – it just goes to show you how much exercise can help you, because I was exactly the same. In that first lockdown – and in fact in the January of the second lockdown – I was really struggling, and walking literally saved me. And you're probably thinking, well, what exercise am I going to get from walking? But just walking in itself is exercise, and you can get quite puffed if you put a bit of effort into it – really pump your arms and pick up the pace a little bit. It's SO good for you.

MAKE AN APPOINTMENT WITH YOURSELF

When I'm really busy with work, and just life in general, the things that really help me, like exercise and mindfulness, fall by the wayside, and before long I can really feel the negative impact.

Think about your hobbies and what you like doing. What are those things that relax you, make you feel good? It doesn't have to be a grand gesture or be super-expensive, it could just be listening to a new podcast or audiobook or going for a walk.

Now put that activity into your diary like you would do with a major work meeting, a parent's evening or your best mate's birthday. Make an appointment for some me time and STICK TO IT.

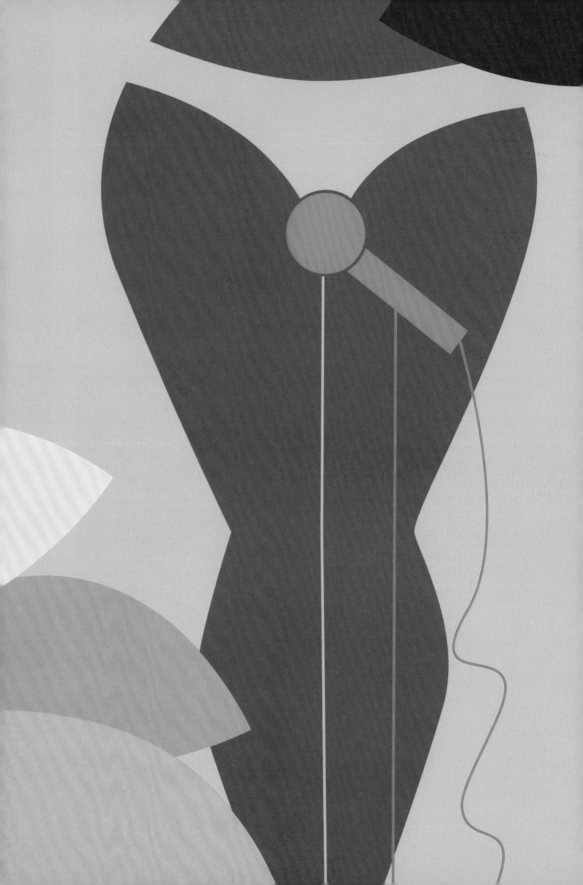

CHAPTER 8

THE DRY VAGINA MONOLOGUES

Vulvovaginal atrophy.

Sounds like your vagina has died and gone to that big arid landscape in the sky, right?

Well, don't panic. We've found the keys. We're going to reopen your shop.

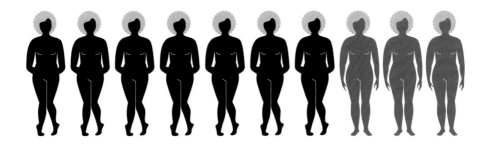

Seven out of ten post-menopausal women suffer from vaginal dryness

Ok, let's talk vaginas. I'm going to talk your vagina, I'm going to talk my vagina; we're specifically talking about dry ones. Dry vag is horrific, I'm afraid. It is as bad as it sounds, although it might not be quite as bad as its medical term, 'vulvovaginal atrophy', which sounds like it's sort of frozen in time, like it's *died*.

But listen to me, loads of us are plagued by this problem, and we mustn't be embarrassed about it – like, *loads and loads* of us, at varying degrees. It is horrible, and we've got to talk about it, because there is an easy, safe fix, ok?

This is a problem that starts during perimenopause and menopause. You know the score: you can get itchy, irritated, inflamed, tight, uncomfortable, sore, angry, downright bloody painful. I bet some of you are crossing your legs just reading this, right?

I know I'm wincing at remembering how painful it was just trying to wipe myself when I was weeing. I used to sit on the loo, and I'd think, *God, why am I sore down there? It's so weird*. And it was because there was no lubrication by my own body, so the loo paper wouldn't slide any more – it kind of got caught. And it was like I was making myself sore. I'd do this little kind of dabby thing instead of a wipe.

Look, I was ashamed, I was embarrassed. I didn't want to talk to anybody about it and I didn't know that it was part of perimenopause. I just thought that I had this weird problem.

I do think it would really, really help if when a doctor is talking to you about your perimenopausal symptoms for them to ask about dry vagina. If any GPs are reading this, it would be super-duper helpful, because we're very good at reeling off all the symptoms that we think you might know, but we'd probably leave off the list any problems with our vaginas. We'd much rather **you** asked **us** if there was a problem with our vagina. We don't even really like talking to each other about our dry vaginas, so we're definitely not going to be madly keen on talking about it to you. So please ask us.

These days, knowing what I know, I wouldn't have a shadow of embarrassment or an ounce of shame talking about it, but I've been perimenopausal – and probably menopausal, I don't know because I've got the Mirena coil – for years now, and I've been wanging on about it forever. But did I tell anybody about it at the time? No. Should I have talked about it? Yes. But why?

Well, over half of post-menopausal women suffer from vaginal dryness[1], and even though it's one of the most common symptoms, it's one of the least talked-about. And we have to change that,

because vaginal dryness can make the simplest things – like exercising, wearing trousers or, God forbid, sitting down – almost impossible. Because it can make sex excruciating. Because it can make even going for a wee feel like torture.

While most symptoms should stop once you reach post-menopause, this one likes to stick around long-term. Your vagina's got its own built-in sound system blasting out Simple Minds' 'Don't You Forget About Me' whenever you unzip your jeans, and no one – no one – needs to hear that!

Then there are related symptoms like UTIs (urinary tract infections), running back and forth to the loo in the middle of the night, and that awful feeling of urgently needing a wee, only to find a dribble comes out. Urgh, I hate that!

Do we talk about these symptoms? No, we don't. That's why I'm calling time on this secretive dry vagina monologue. What we need instead is a vagina DIALOGUE, to bring this problem out into the open and face it front-bum-on.

If these symptoms sound all too familiar, you need to know that it's not ok to put up with it, and there are ways you can deal with it effectively, and for good. HRT vaginal oestrogen is cheap, effective and it does NOT carry the risks thought to be associated with systemic HRT.

---

[1] Women's Health Concern (2020). 'Vaginal dryness', www.womens-health-concern.org/help-and-advice/factsheets/vaginal-dryness/

Three super-important things to remember:

You aren't the only one.

You have NOTHING to be embarrassed about.

Vaginal dryness isn't something you have to live with. It is totally treatable. You have options, and we're going to give them to you right now.

FANNY, MINGE, LADY GARDEN... DO YOU KNOW YOUR VULVA FROM YOUR CLITORIS?

Before we get stuck in, let's just pause and make sure we're all on the same page when it comes to terminology.

Lots of people use the terms vagina and vulva interchangeably, but they are completely different organs. A 2021 study[2] found that almost forty per cent of Brits mislabelled the clitoris on a diagram, half didn't label the labia correctly and only eighteen per cent knew where the perineum was.

Fanny, minge or lady garden – does it really matter what you call it? Of course not. I'm not saying we all need a PhD in pubic studies or must all start playing a game of pin the tail on the vulva (bad idea – *please* don't do that). But *knowing* and using the proper names can really help you communicate your symptoms at appointments, pinpoint problems and get the treatment you need.

So, no laughing at the back, and repeat after me...

The **vulva** is the catch-all term for the external organs you can see, including the opening of the vagina, inner and outer lips (labia) and the clitoris.

The **vagina** is the tunnel of love inside the labia (about 8cm long, fact-fans).

WHAT'S HAPPENED TO MY VAGINA?

Oestrogen is responsible for keeping our vulvas and vaginas happy, healthy and in good working order. It helps keep the tissues lubricated and plump and the muscles stretchy, supple and strong.

When oestrogen levels fall during perimenopause and menopause, those structures lose their strength, tissues become thin and more fragile, and the muscles lose their strength and stretchiness.

That's what causes the burning and irritation that I found when dabbing myself after a wee, but for some women it can be so extreme that they can barely sit or have clothing touching it.

So many of you were really candid about your struggles with vaginal dryness, which I know from personal experience isn't the easiest thing to talk about.

But it's so important that we do.

---

[2] D. El-Hamamsy et al. (2021), 'Public understanding of female genital anatomy and pelvic organ prolapse (POP); a questionnaire-based pilot study', International Urogynecology Journal, Doi.org/10.1007/s00192-021-04727-9.

'I couldn't carry on being in so much pain.' — Alison

Among those to share her story was sixty-year-old Alison, who has been plagued by vaginal dryness for the past decade, along with low sex drive, crippling anxiety and panic attacks. She convinced herself it was just cystitis, but every time she had a urine sample taken the results nearly always came back negative. Alison did some more of her own research and came to the realisation the symptoms she'd been living with for the last decade sounded very much like vaginal dryness.

Vaginal dryness has been an utter nightmare and at times has caused me to think of taking my own life.

During the decade of suffering with this I have been in so much pain and discomfort that walking, bending, sitting and even lying in bed has been unbearable at times.

Then finally my doctor suggested I had a cystoscopy [a procedure to look inside the bladder using a thin camera to check for problems in the bladder or urethra] but they couldn't find anything wrong.

I was determined to get to the bottom of the cause of my problem. Then just by chance I started following Liz Earle, who spoke a lot about her experience of the menopause and how she wanted to help other women going through the same.

I came to realise that I may have to consider taking HRT. I had always been against HRT but I knew in my heart that I couldn't possibly carry on life being in so much pain. My family were also suffering knowing I was so unhappy.

Last year I politely told my doctor that I wanted to start HRT. Now I realise it was one of the best decisions that I have taken. It took about six months for my symptoms to improve but I now feel amazing. The quality of my life and my family's life are both so much better.

Oh my goodness Alison, I loved this story. Firstly, because it is SO important to talk about this stuff. Secondly, because you mention Liz Earle, who is such an amazing menopause warrior and has done such fantastic things for women. I love the fact that **her** speaking out about **her** issue helped **you**, and now **you** speaking out about **your** issue is going to help so many women. This is what I love: women supporting other women; it's fantastic. And I'm so pleased that the quality of your life, and your family's life, is so much better.

SORENESS, TAMPON TROUBLE AND ELECTRIC SHOCKS: TELL-TALE SIGNS OF VAGINAL DRYNESS ... AND SOME SURPRISING ONES, TOO

Some of the most common symptoms include:

→ Soreness

→ Redness

→ Itch and burning

→ Inflammation/swelling

→ Pain during sex

→ Dryness before and during sex

→ Pain when having a cervical smear

A tampon falling out can often be one of the early signs that you've developed vaginal dryness. This happens because it's more difficult to place your tampon high enough up and the muscles inside the vagina are less strong.

Those thinning tissues don't just affect inside of the vagina: your labia, clitoris and the opening to the vagina can all become thin and split. And while most will notice a lack of lubrication, atrophy can actually lead to more discharge than before.

A lesser-known symptom is electric shock sensation, which has been appropriately nicknamed 'lightning fanny' by one of Dr Naomi's patients.

VAGINAL DRYNESS IS NOT THE SAME AS THRUSH

Many women often mistake vaginal dryness for thrush, especially if they've had thrush in the past.

It's easy to see why, because some of the symptoms, such as the soreness and the irritation, are the same.

Ask yourself:

→ Is it painful to sit, exercise or wear tight clothing?

→ Have you recently had a smear test? Smear tests can be uncomfortable, but they shouldn't be painful.

→ Do you have soreness, lack of lubrication or pain during sex?

→ Has your vulva changed in appearance?

→ If you are on HRT, and your other symptoms have improved, vaginal dryness can persist. If this is the case, please discuss with your doctor. Many find that adding a topical oestrogen product (cream, gel, pessary or ring) to your routine is often needed.

NO MORE SHAME, NO MORE EMBARRASSMENT

While a lot of women will quite happily talk openly about their hot flushes, when it comes to vaginal symptoms, that's a closed book – and that's understandable. Think back to those hushed sex ed classes at school, and the fact that the dolls we played with as children didn't have any genitalia. Talking about vulvas and vaginas just wasn't what 'polite' girls did. And for some parts of society, it still isn't.

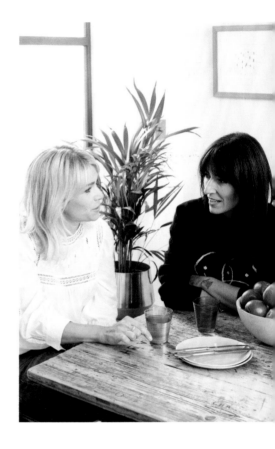

That has to change. Vaginal dryness isn't the sort of problem that will go away by itself. If you have these symptoms, please go and get them checked out so you and your doctor can come up with a proper treatment to suit you.

Doctors are used to seeing vulvas of all shapes and sizes, so there really is no need to feel embarrassed.

Vaginal dryness is totally treatable, but it needs the *right sort* of treatment, long term.

If you want to read more on the subject, then check out *Me & My Menopausal Vagina* by Jane Lewis.

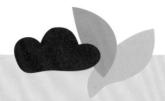

NOW I KNOW WHAT THE PROBLEM IS – HOW DO I FIX IT? DR NAOMI'S GUIDE TO TREATMENTS

Here's an outline of the prescription and over-the-counter treatments that can help banish these horrible symptoms and let you get back to living your life.

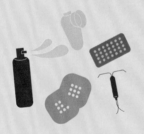

SYSTEMIC HRT

Systemic HRT can be an effective treatment for vaginal dryness, along with other symptoms. You should expect dryness symptoms to start to improve within a few months.

However, HRT may not be enough for everyone, so here are some targeted treatments to tackle vaginal dryness.

TOPICAL OESTROGEN – CREAMS AND GELS

Known as topical oestrogen because you use them directly on the area, these treatments will replace the oestrogen, give your tissues a chance to repair and generally improve symptoms.

Creams and gels are applied to the skin of the vulva and vagina. Typically, you would apply a cream or gel every day for the first few weeks, then once, twice or three times a week thereafter on direction of a nurse or doctor.

How do I use it?

You can use it one of two ways: insert the cream directly into your vagina with an applicator – most users prefer to do this at bedtime so it stays in place while you are sleeping. Or you can also use your fingertips to apply cream on and around your vulva. The gel comes with an applicator, or use your fingertips.

Pros

+ The applicator can reduce mess.

+ You can also use it on and around your vulva, so it's good for external symptoms too.

Cons

– It still can be a bit messy!

– Currently only available on prescription, but this may change.

– Some women find them locally irritating.

VAGINAL OESTROGEN PESSARY

These are typically used every day for the first two weeks and twice a week after that.

How do I use it?

Some pessaries come with a disposable applicator to insert a pessary into your vagina. There are also lower-dose pessaries that look like little bullets and don't require an applicator.

Pros

+ Some people prefer pessaries as they are less messy than cream.

Cons

– Unlike cream and gels, you can only use pessaries directly in the vagina.

– The non-applicator pessaries in particular can produce a discharge when they dissolve.

– Some women find them locally irritating.

PRASTERONE INTRAROSA

This is a pessary that contains Prasterone DHEA. It works by being converted into oestrogen and androgens which then act upon the local tissues.

How do I use it?

You can use it with or without an applicator.

OESTROGEN RINGS

These rings are placed inside the vagina and the oestrogen is released gradually over three months.

How do I use it?

These are soft, flexible silicon rings that you simply put inside your vagina, or a health professional can do this for you on your first try.

Pros

+ You can pop it in and forget about it.

+ Remove before sex or leave in.

+ An alternative to creams, gels and pessaries, and not as messy.

Cons

- Needs to be replaced every three months.

- Some women find them fiddly.

SENSHIO

Senshio is an oral tablet. It is indicated for the treatment of moderate to severe symptomatic vulvar and vaginal atrophy (VVA) in post-menopausal women who are not candidates for local vaginal oestrogen therapy. The active substance in Senshio, ospemifene, is a selective oestrogen receptor modulator (SERM). This means that it acts in the same way as oestrogen in some tissues in the body such as the vagina and so helps to reduce symptoms of vulvovaginal atrophy.

WHAT ABOUT NON-HORMONE TREATMENTS?

There are some over-the-counter products that you can use alongside HRT or topical oestrogen, or just on their own if you are unable to or don't want to use HRT. These treatments can help make you more comfortable. They won't replace the hormones in the way HRT and topical oestrogen does.

Vaginal moisturisers will help restore moisture, soothe tissues and alleviate irritation and burning. The best ones are also balanced to match the natural pH and osmolality of the vagina.[3] Like oestrogen cream or gel, you can use an applicator to insert the moisturiser into the vagina, or your fingertips to use on and around the vulva. You can use the moisturiser daily for the first week or

[3] N. Potter, N. Panay (2021) 'Vaginal lubricants and moisturizers: a review into use, efficacy, and safety', Climacteric, Doi: 10.1080/13697137.2020.1820478.

so, and then see if you can reduce to a few times a week thereafter depending on how severe your symptoms are.

Lubricants applied to the vulva and vagina can be used just before sex to lubricate the vagina. Choose one with a pH of between 3.8 and 4.5.

Try to avoid products containing ingredients like parabens, nonoxynol and chlorhexidine.

USING TOPICAL OESTROGEN? WHY THE PATIENT INFORMATION LEAFLET CAN BE MISLEADING

When you get your prescription, whether it's a cream, pessary or gel, it will come with a concertina-like patient information leaflet – or the patient misinformation leaflet, as I like to call it.

Often, alongside the usage instructions are a raft of health warnings. But these warnings are scary and misleading, because the risks listed apply to systemic HRT rather than topical HRT.

The truth is that these products are extremely safe to use in practically every scenario:

→ Vaginal oestrogen **does not** carry the same risks of usual HRT.

→ It does **not** increase the risk of breast cancer.

→ It does **not** increase the risk of clot.

→ You **do not** have to stop using it after a few years, which is so important, as dryness often persists into your post-menopause years.

Topical oestrogen is safe. It works and it can be used almost indefinitely.

OTHER TOP TIPS

→ Perfumed body washes can make irritation worse, it is best to use warm water when washing.

→ You can ask your doctor to prescribe an emollient – moisturising treatments that cover the skin with a protective film to trap in moisture and soothe sore skin.

→ Avoid tight clothing until you get the symptoms under control.

Up in the night for a wee AGAIN?

Can't get the key in the door FAST ENOUGH?

Yet another UTI?

Leaking when you LAUGH or SNEEZE?

PEE, INFECTIONS AND YOUR PELVIC FLOOR

There are many urinary issues that you need to look out for.

. . . . . .

'I've had UTIs for a decade.' — Helen

I've suffered from water infections for the last ten years. I've had ultrasound scans and a camera to check everything is ok inside. I've had six months of antibiotics at a low dose, and I am still suffering. I'm fifty-five now and I'm convinced it's all to do with the menopause...

Thanks Helen, it does sound menopausal to me and I really hope you've got this sorted now.

Oestrogen not only keeps our vulvas and vagina happy and healthy, but our urinary system too. Oestrogen keeps the muscles in our pelvic floor taut and strong (I bet you're doing pelvic floor exercises right now? Yeah, me too), and this in turn keeps our uterus, bladder and bowel where they should be.

Not only that, but a strong pelvic floor plays a big part in a satisfying sex life: one of the deeper layers of muscles in the pelvic floor plays a big part in sensation and strength of orgasms.

But when oestrogen is depleted, these muscles become weaker. Not only that, but we have oestrogen receptors all along our urinary tract that are super-sensitive to any hormonal changes, while the lining of our bladders and urethras (the tube that carries pee from the bladder to outside your body) thins.

This can lead to symptoms like:

→ Stress incontinence – leaking when you laugh, sneeze or cough, or pick up something heavy.

→ Frequent urge to pee, particularly at night.

→ Urge incontinence – when you desperately need to wee and can't make it to the toilet in time.

About one in three women are living with urinary incontinence.[4] Ok, it's not life-threatening, but there is a perception that the odd bit of leakage when you laugh, or needing to have tactical pees 'just in case' you get caught short is something you have to put up with after having kids or going through menopause. Nothing could be further from the truth, and these symptoms can make you really miserable and affect your quality of life.

The menopause can change the pH balance in the vagina, it can also make you more susceptible to UTIs and other infections, which can be debilitating and hard to treat. If they continue to go untreated you can end up with chronic infection, which can be life-altering.

SIGNS YOU HAVE A UTI INCLUDE:

→ Needing to pass urine urgently.

→ Pain or burning whilst passing urine.

→ The desire to pass urine, and only small amounts are then passed.

→ Cloudy, offensive or blood-stained urine.

→ Lower abdominal or back pain.

→ A fever.

'I lost count at twelve UTIs.' — Sharon

Just ask Sharon. Her menopause was fairly uneventful until she started to be plagued by recurrent UTIs. She first noticed pain during a routine smear test. Eventually, Sharon turned to a nutritionist, followed a sugar-free diet and tried various supplements, which helped but was difficult to maintain. The UTIs started to creep back, until eventually she got the help she needed.

The nurse struggled to do my smear as the pain was excruciating. This took me by surprise; I'd never had problems before. I wondered why, but no reason was mentioned. I wasn't sexually active so I just tried to ignore the situation, but when I exercised, particularly when I did yoga, it felt very uncomfortable, with a deep burning sensation.

---

[4] NHS England 'Excellence in Continence Care' (2018) https://www.england.nhs.uk/wp-content/uploads/2018/07/excellence-in-continence-care.pdf

Six months later I had a UTI after a long-haul flight. Then another and another... I lost count after twelve UTIs and three kidney infections. I went to see my doctor, whose only advice was to wipe from front to back after going to the toilet and always have a shower before sex. Er... hello, I'm fifty-eight, I know how to shower and I understand basic hygiene!

Then a helpful female GP said they could be linked to vaginal atrophy, and that vaginal pessaries may help. I started them straight away and OMG the difference was amazing. I had suffered

for two years not realising the knock-on effect my lack of oestrogen was having. I wish I'd looked into this earlier.

I don't like to think of all the antibiotics I've had to take over the years because of the UTIs – before I had UTIs I rarely needed them. If only my GP or nurse had correlated the menopause with UTIs – it would have been sorted years ago.

'Why does nobody talk about it?' — Sarah

And it's not just UTIs that you have all been struggling with. Sarah suffers from vulvodynia, or persistent unexplained pain in the vulva that can be caused by hormone changes.

It took me years to get a diagnosis. That was after years of suffering and feelings of constant thrush, cystitis and pain flare-ups, anxiety and feelings of going mad.

Why does nobody talk about it??

'The itching is indescribable.' — Claire

Claire was diagnosed with a skin condition called lichen sclerosus that can cause patches of white skin on the genitals. The condition had been dormant for many years, but became worse during menopause, making her life a 'living hell'.

Most days I wanted to tear myself apart with the itching. My sleep was affected as the itching at night was so much worse; my sex life was non-existent. I hadn't attributed it to menopause until I went to see a life-changing GP who listened to me whilst I was balling my eyes out.

The intense itching and thinning of the skin is indescribable. After being examined, my GP went on to tell me how I had vaginal atrophy and thinning. I had small fissures and breaks on the skin surface, along with blisters, which had been causing my discomfort.

Her answer immediately was HRT... she went on to explain that the condition had become so much worse due to the depletion of all the hormones I had in my body prior to going through the menopause. I cried my eyes out again at the relief that someone was listening.

I have now been on HRT for two years and although this condition is something *I have to 'manage', the symptoms are considerably reduced due to taking HRT... there were times that I questioned how I could bear living with the effects of this condition for the rest of my life.*

Sharon, Sarah and Claire, thank you very much for sharing those stories, because it is really important that women hear about all the different ways that menopause and perimenopause can affect our vaginas and our waterworks. But I'm so pleased that we all seem to be talking about it, because these stories will definitely help women go and seek out the support and treatment that they need. Because, as we've read, this is a treatment that you can carry on for the rest of your life, and will give you a beautiful, fully working, squishy, lubed-up vagina.

The other really scary thing is how we have heard from Claire and other women in this book that they have often wondered if they can actually carry on living with some of their conditions for the rest of their lives. This is unacceptable.

WHAT CAN I DO ABOUT IT?

The good news is that there are options to ease these symptoms and make daily life a lot more comfortable.

→ **Replace hormones:** Systemic, topical HRT, or both, will replace the hormones.

→ **If you think you have a UTI, see a doctor:** Don't be tempted to self-medicate. You might need antibiotics to clear the infection.

→ **Bladder training:** Try and pass urine only when you really need to, rather than just in case. This retrains the bladder into knowing when it is full.

→ **Supplements:** D-Mannose is a supplement that can reduce the risk of UTIs and can help to prevent bacteria from sticking to the walls of the urinary tract and causing infection.

→ **Pelvic floor problems:** Ask to be referred to a specialist or a women's health physiotherapist.

'The lights have gone out on our sex life.' — Gemma

Gemma is in menopause after treatment for Stage 3 cervical cancer. When she shared her story she was waiting to be seen by an HRT specialist, six months after finishing treatment.

Getting diagnosed with cervical cancer was hard because I felt the GP wasn't listening to me when I was saying my bleeding wasn't normal. He hasn't spoken to me about the menopause or HRT and I'm waiting on a hospital referral to come through.

At my first appointment to talk about treatment after my diagnosis, menopause was just a bullet-point note in the possible side-effects after treatment, that's it. After treatment, I was, I am, a complete mess.

As well as recovering from radiotherapy and chemotherapy I started waking up in pools of sweat. Hot flushes are so intense, I'm needing to strip off as much as possible. I feel completely alone, none of my friends understand.

My partner is hanging on in there, but the lights have gone out on our sex life. I have no drive, using dilators after treatment hurts, then having a wee hurts after I use one, so the thought of sex is as far back in my mind as possible.

I'm gaining weight but not eating massive amounts because I've lost my appetite for food and alcohol after treatment.

I used to be quite fit, I loved running, but I have no motivation to get going, I have aches and pains in my hips and legs.

I'm becoming very forgetful and I'm struggling with anxiety and brain fog. I started talking about my problems on Instagram and I recently set up a new page on there so I could talk more about what I was going through; I want to talk about the cervical cancer, menopause and surrogacy. I've been thrown into a world I don't know or understand with no help or warning on how badly my life was going to change.

Gemma, thank you so much for letting us use this in the book – and I really, really hope that you are reading this and it will help you understand what you're going through. And maybe you can seek some help with some of your symptoms, because you can definitely, definitely alleviate some of them with some of the things that we have talked about here, and I really hope that they work for you.

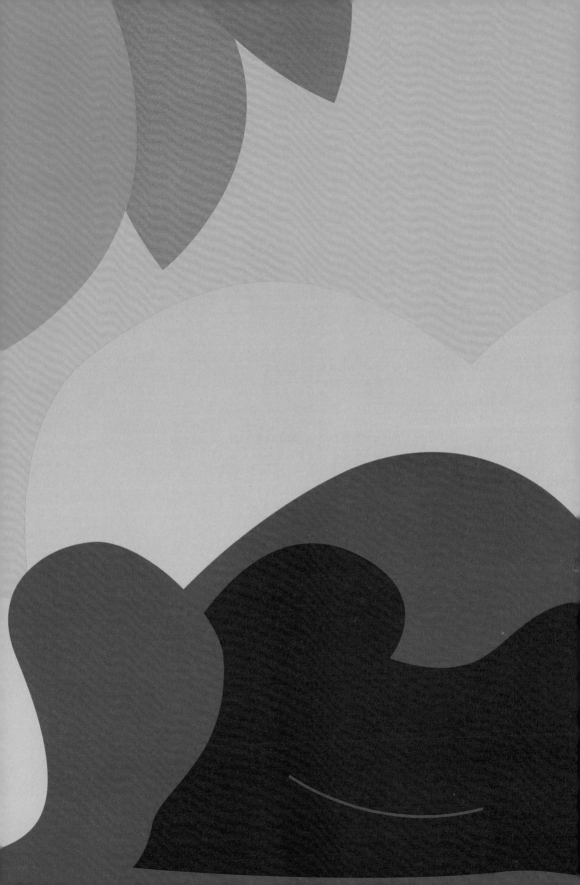

CHAPTER 9

FEELING FRISKY: WHY GREAT SEX DOESN'T STOP AT THE MENOPAUSE

'I want the old, sexy me back.'

'I told my doctor about my vaginal dryness...they told me to USE IT OR LOSE IT.'

'The lights have gone out on our sex life.'

'Sex is different now...but it's BETTER.'

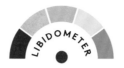

84% of perimenopausal and menopausal women think having an active sex life is important[1]

But 80% said the perimenopause or menopause had affected their sex drive

Let's not beat around the bush (sorry); menopause can wreak havoc with your sex life.

The hormone crash, the soreness, the 'I've been up since 6am and I just can't be bothered' feeling when your other half nudges you and suggests a cheeky roll in the hay.

So many women tell me their sex life is MIA and they aren't sure they will ever get their mojo back. I've been there. I felt spectacularly unattractive during my sweaty nights and my sore, dry vagina and my dry skin, and my brain fog – none of this made me feel sexy. But I want you all to know that you can and will have mind-blowing, swinging-from-the-chandeliers sex during and

after menopause (if you want it) and I've got just the woman to help show us how: the amazing Samantha Evans, whom I absolutely adore. She's a former nurse and founder of Jo Divine, which, if you want to buy any kind of sex toy, clothing, lubricant – anything – is a fantastic website to go to. She's an all-round sexpert. She is so knowledgeable, but especially for perimenopausal and menopausal women, and later in this chapter she's got some fabulous tips to get your rocks off in the bedroom.

You might remember Sam from my documentary. Her advice was *so* good that you guys cleared out her website within hours of the programme airing. I went on her website just to have a look – obviously for work purposes– but

---

[1] G.P Cumming, H.D Currie, R Moncur, A.J Lee (2009), 'Web-based survey on the effect of menopause on women's libido in a computer-literate population', Menopause International, 15(1), pp.8-12]

203

literally nothing: everything had run out of stock. So I knew I just had to make her part of this book.

So get ready for Sam's menopause sex 101, from the saucy kit you need on standby at your bedside table, the best communication tips for partners and the benefits of getting your self-love on.

Plus we'll be hearing your stories on how menopause has affected your sex life, including one woman who swears it actually saved her marriage.

How can I get the intimacy back? Do I really need lube? What sex toy should I buy? And how do I tell my partner what I really, *really* want? Maybe you're desperate to reclaim your sex life, or just want some no-nonsense advice on how to keep things fresh. Whatever you need, you'll find the answers here.

NOT TONIGHT, DARLING: HOW MENOPAUSE HITS YOUR LIBIDO

Sore down below? Low self-esteem? Zero interest in your partner? Painful sex?

You definitely aren't alone. So many of you shared your stories of how the menopause has sent your sex drive through the floor.

'The old Diane has gone and I'm not liking it one bit.' — Diane

Diane started HRT three months ago but says her mood and libido still haven't improved.

Bang out of the blue, about a year ago now, tiredness, dryness down below, lethargy, zero libido, brain fog, weight gain, irritability.

I'm on HRT but not feeling much benefit. I try to eat healthily and walk daily when I can ... I feel old and sad at times, no longer sexy or desired, and my marriage has suffered because of menopause.

Sometimes I feel I'm going mad. I have even had suicidal thoughts and that was never me, I'm normally upbeat and the life and soul of the party. It's like the old

Diane has gone and I'm not liking it one bit. I want the old me back, the sexy, confident lady with no cares.

Diane, **please** go back to visit your doctor to see if there's anything they can do to help. It might be worth talking to them about your dosage or about trying testosterone as well.

'I'm in libido limbo – what happens now??' — Jane

Jane, who is smart, successful and wants to have sex, has been on the receiving end of some pretty unhelpful advice from her doctor.

When I asked my female GP for advice about my vaginal dryness she said something along the lines of 'use it or lose it'. She mentioned atrophy, but no solutions. The nurse suggested 'lubing up to the max'.

My last sexual encounter came as a bit of a shock: I had sex with a new chap and it only lasted a few seconds. I'd never had a problem with dryness in the past, but it wasn't actually the best position for me and I was nowhere near stimulated enough. In response to the incredible pain, and out of frustration, I blurted out 'oh, rubbish', which killed the mood somewhat.

The chap thought it was a slur on his performance (which was rather speedy, to be honest). He said his performance had never been rated that badly before, and, unsurprisingly, we never saw each other again.

I know it sounds like a funny scene from a film, but this is me, a real person with a dry vagina. I'm scared to enter into a relationship: I want to have sex, but I'm afraid of being rejected.

I enjoy masturbation, but I miss another person's skin, touch, voice and support... oh my, I'm crying writing this bit. I have been in two long-term relationships and had a few flings in between. I am only fifty-seven. A homeowner, successful in my work, funny, attractive, sore down below... I am in libido limbo and what happens now?

Hey Jane, thanks for your story. I do hope you read Chapter 8 about vaginal dryness, because there is an easy fix for that, but libido limbo is not good: please keep reading.

GETTING YOUR MOJO BACK

In most cases, there is no one set reason why sex drive can suffer during menopause. Here are a few of the culprits:

Vaginal dryness: Sore and painful, it's a huge barrier to a healthy and fulfilling sex life. Your vagina is less lubricated, more susceptible to infection, and dryness can also affect the clitoris, too.

UTIs and other infections: Likewise, the oestrogen drop can also trigger similar changes in the urethra and leave you at risk of UTIs.

Other physical symptoms: Hot flushes and night sweats or weight gain can really affect your self-esteem.

Relationship problems: Often work and home stress, plus relationship tension, can spill over into your sex life. A lack of communication or feeling irritable, frustrated or exasperated with your partner is hardly the recipe for a night of passion. Add overwhelming tiredness, crippling headaches and aches and pains into the mix, and it is no wonder sex might be the last thing on your mind.

WHAT CAN I DO ABOUT IT?

The first step in rediscovering your sex drive is addressing hormone issues. The first line of treatment would normally be HRT. This will help with symptoms like fatigue, hot flushes and low mood and this in itself can get your libido back fairly quickly.

If you suffer from vaginal dryness or recurrent UTIs you may benefit from a topical oestrogen. Applying oestrogen products directly to your vagina and vulva can ease symptoms and re-oestrogenise the tissues to enable them to become soft, supple and lubricated again.

There's a variety of types to choose from, including gel, creams, tablets and rings, and which one you opt for depends on personal preference and what fits in with your lifestyle (see pages 188–189).

Topical oestrogen carries practically no risk because it delivers oestrogen directly to the vagina and there is minimal absorption. You can use it for as long as you are feeling the benefits, because it is safe to use indefinitely.

There are also non-hormonal treatments such as water- or oil-based lubricants and moisturisers that can improve dryness and make sex more comfortable.

Once you are established on HRT, if your libido is still low, then testosterone may help. Returning testosterone to normal levels can help increase libido, improve sexual function and orgasms.

Testosterone can be particularly important if you have had an early or surgical menopause, because symptoms of testosterone deficiency tend to be more profound. A surgical menopause is a menopause that occurs immediately during surgery, when a sudden loss of testosterone can be very apparent.

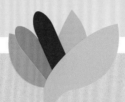

MENOPAUSE SEX 101, BY SAMANTHA EVANS

I'm Samantha Evans, former nurse and co-founder of sex toy retailer Jo Divine.

My work revolves around helping people have better sex, because I know first-hand how much it matters.

In my twenties and thirties, I was plagued by thrush, bacterial vaginosis, recurrent cystitis and UTIs that led to vaginismus – a painful condition where the vagina muscles tighten up when penetration is attempted.

Relying on poor sexual lubricants, many of which are still available on the market and are often recommended by healthcare professionals, ruined my vaginal health, and my sex life.

So over the next few pages I'll be sharing my tips on how you can reclaim your libido and start enjoying some of the best sex of your life.

TIME TO RECLAIM YOUR INTIMATE HEALTH

Topical oestrogen can be a game-changer when it comes to enjoying pleasurable sex and preventing issues like irritation and recurrent infections like thrush.

I personally use pessaries that I pop inside my vagina three times a week, and I have to say it has transformed my vagina and bladder health, in addition to making sex feel even more pleasurable.

And while many of us are prepared to part with £££s for moisturisers that leave our skin soft and supple, little thought is given to how to keep the skin inside our vagina and our vulva happy.

But good intimate health goes hand in hand with our sexual pleasure, particularly during and after menopause.

YOUR VAGINA DOESN'T NEED TO SMELL LIKE ROSES

Newsflash: our wonderful, clever vaginas are actually self-cleaning. Using unnecessary washes and treatments destroys the friendly bacteria in them, which we need to maintain the pH balance to prevent conditions such as thrush or bacterial vaginosis and to help with vaginal lubrication.

If you experience vaginal dryness, tightness, shrinking, soreness, itching or recurrent infections, talk to your doctor.

The tissues in the vagina are delicate, so treat them with care. Ditch the heavily perfumed washes, bubble bath, shower gels, bath bombs (or, as they are known in my house, thrush bombs). You should only be using water, or ask your doctor to prescribe a gentle emollient if you really feel like you need to wash with a product.

WHY A GOOD LUBE IS YOUR NEW BEST FRIEND

Some people will baulk at the idea of using lube, they should be instantly wet at the slightest touch. Lube isn't just for vaginal dryness: it's great used with sex toys and can help take sexual pleasure to new heights – whatever your age. We have customers well into their nineties!

GLITTER, GLYCERIN ... AND CHILLI: INGREDIENTS TO AVOID

It pays to do your homework before you buy – and that means more than a quick scan of the chemist aisle at the local supermarket or high-street chemist. Think of yourself as an 'ingredient detective': a good sexual lubricant is a real investment, so it absolutely pays to take your time and have a good read of the ingredients.

Ones to watch out for include:

→ **Glycerin** – can cause thrush.

→ **Propylene glycol** – that stinging feeling when you first try using a lube? Often that will be down to propylene glycol.

→ **Parabens** – preservatives used in so many products, including those designed for intimate use, but again, they can irritate the sensitive skin. KY Jelly, often recommended by doctors and other healthcare professionals, contains parabens and glycerine.

→ **Alcohol** – very drying to the skin and even more so to the delicate tissues of our vaginas and vulvas.

→ **Dyes and perfumes** – these might make the lube look and smell nice, but neither are good news for your vaginal or vulval health.

→ **'Tingling' or 'cooling' lubricants** – some people use warming and cooling lubricants to enhance sexual pleasure, but I would exercise caution. Often the tingling effect is caused by menthol or chilli, which can be damaging to the delicate tissues of our genitals.

→ **Glitter** – also a definite no-no, unless you want to be picking bits of glitter out of your nether regions.

Just because a product is slippery does not mean it's suitable for sex. Please, please, please keep vegetable oils for your salad, baby oil for your body and petroleum jelly for your lips. These products are not designed for sexual use, many contain irritating ingredients and can cause infections, and they can damage sex toys and condoms, too.

SO, WHAT LUBE SHOULD I USE?

The good news is that there are now lots of good-quality, skin-safe lubricants on the market.

→ **Water-based lubricants** are the closest to your own natural lubrication, they are easy to wash off, can be used for any sexual activity, and with condoms and any sex toy material, including silicone toys.

→ **Oil-based lubricants** are longer-lasting but aren't suitable for use with latex condoms.

→ **Silicone lubricants** have a major advantage in that a little goes a long way, but they aren't suitable for use with silicone sex toys.

MOISTURISE YOUR VAGINA AND VULVA? ARE YOU MAD????*

(*IT'S ACTUALLY A VERY GOOD IDEA)

The tissues of your vulva and vagina age like the rest of your body and need TLC to keep them happy and healthy so you can keep enjoying great sex.

So what should you use to moisturise your vulva and vagina? Ingredients matter, so just as with lubricant, you need to play ingredient detective again, avoiding irritating ingredients such as glycerin, parabens, perfumes, dyes, alcohol and petroleum jelly.

Again, it pays to think before you buy. Grabbing the cheapest product from the shelf may leave you with irritation or even an infection. And if your doctor prescribes or recommends a vaginal moisturiser, make a point of asking what the ingredients are.

WAYS TO SPICE THINGS UP

Don't let boredom and routine get in the way of having great sex. Sex doesn't need to be a huge performance: look at the ways in which you can spice it up, be it with a good lube and sex toys, booking a night away somewhere, or just enjoying kissing and cuddling like you did at the start of your relationship. Sex is so much more than penetration, so get creative and discover different sexual sensations. You might find you love to be spanked or be the spanker, you enjoy tapping into your dominant side or that you love giving and receiving oral sex.

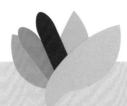

MASTURBATION AND MENOPAUSE: SAM'S SEVEN REASONS TO GET YOUR SELF-LOVE ON

Many people think that sexual satisfaction involves being in a relationship, but not every aspect of your sex life requires a partner.

Whether you're single or in a long-term relationship, indulging in a bit of 'me' time has a raft of benefits.

→ **It kickstarts your libido** – the more you masturbate, the more pleasurable it will feel and you'll want to keep doing it – which in turn helps to boost your libido.

→ **Stress-busting** – orgasming releases endorphins and serotonin, which can reduce stress and balance your mood.

→ **Helps you sleep** – the endorphin release can lower blood pressure and induce a state of relaxation to promote a good night's sleep – much more exciting than a mug of cocoa!

→ **Natural painkiller** – masturbation is probably the last thing on your mind when you are on your period, but orgasming can help relieve cramping from periods by encouraging blood flow to the pelvic area.

→ **Boosts your chances of enjoying an orgasm during penetrative sex** – exploring what works for you helps you be more assertive about what works for you with a partner.

→ **Safe** – there's no risk of getting a sexually transmitted infection or becoming pregnant.

→ And, above all, it is bloody good **FUN!**

WHY YOU NEED A SEX TOY IN YOUR LIFE

A good sex toy is essential when you are menopausal. They are a great way to get warmed up, to boost your arousal or add into your sex play. Some toys can also help with menopausal symptoms, such as vaginal tightness, painful sex and decreased sexual sensation, and offer enjoyment for non-penetrative sex.

Sex toy design has come a long way since the days of *Sex and the City* and the Rampant Rabbit (made from jelly-like material). These days there is a whole range of cleverly designed products with powerful motors, creative technology and skin-safe materials to experiment with and enjoy.

Whether you're a sex toy virgin or a pro, there'll be something to suit you. And if you are unsure what to try, here are some suggestions to get you started.

Bullet vibrators – smaller than the average vibrator and get their name from the sleek design, but can still pack a powerful punch with a range of pulsating patterns. Designed for external use with a tapered tip for pinpoint stimulation, bullet vibrators are a great toy for beginners and their discreet size makes them a great choice when travelling.

Classic vibrators – designed for both vaginal and clitoral play and come in all sorts of shapes, sizes, colours, textures and vibration speeds. They can deliver both vaginal and clitoral stimulation. Many have tapered heads for pinpoint clitoral stimulation, while a powerful motor sends a strong vibration along the shaft for an intense vaginal sensation.

Air pulse clitoral stimulators – many people assume that vibrators are all designed to be put inside you, but a really popular toy is the LELO Sona 2, which is the 'game-changer' I chatted about with Davina in her documentary. This toy absorbs sonic waves and pulses and transmits them back to the internal and external parts of the clitoris. It feels amazing, and is perfect if you find it hard to orgasm through penetration alone.

This picture is of me discussing vibrators. That's how happy I look when I am discussing sex toys.

I feel like we are on the cusp of a sexual revolution and that women are no longer embarrassed to be talking about sex or sex toys. There are wonderful celebrities who have completely normalised this – Lily Allen famously co-designed her own vibrator. We're now all discussing sex toys, or vibrators, or ways that we can enjoy sex together in a much more open way. This isn't to say that I'm promoting sleeping with thousands of people! I'm just saying that for women, this is quite a new and refreshing concept. We are all really being given permission to now enjoy sex, whereas we were previously always told to just put up and shut up.

This is a revolution. So, if there's something that you've discovered and works for you, tell your friends about it. Tell everyone about it. We all deserve to enjoy ourselves, with a partner or solo.

I mean, this is also a new concept. I know men that didn't realise women masturbate. But hello, we do, and we should. And it's a fantastic, cheap and safe way of having a really nice time.

We should be proud of being sexual creatures and live long, prosperous, happy, sexy lives.

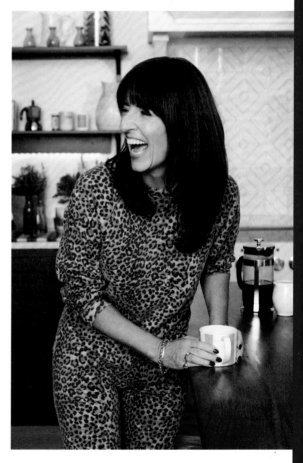

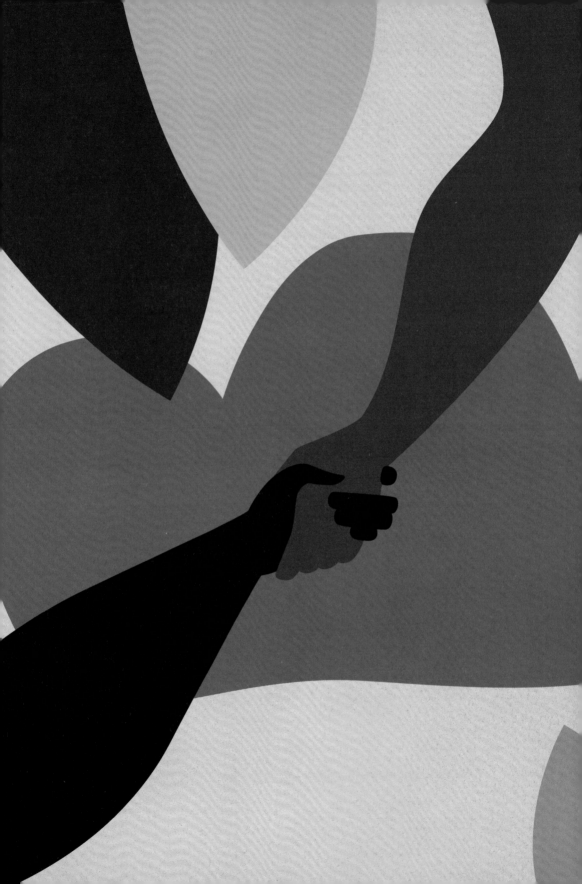

CHAPTER 10

BATTEN DOWN THE HATCHES: HOW TO MENOPAUSE-PROOF YOUR RELATIONSHIPS AND MAKE THEM STRONGER

'My kids have been walking on EGGSHELLS.'

'Got asked into my boss's office ... thought I was getting FIRED.'

'My body ached, my head ached, my heart ached and my relationship with my husband and kids was suffering, but I tried to be STOIC and CARRY ON.'

Let's talk relationships. Let's talk about *all* relationships – not just those with our partners, but also with our children, our families, our friends, our bosses, our colleagues – with everybody. And also, especially, the relationship with ourselves, in terms of how we cope with what's going on in all the other relationships.

Sometimes things can be so difficult that our self-esteem can hit the floor, because it just feels like we are constantly pushing away everybody we love and care about with our behaviour, and yet we seem to be completely powerless to stop this.

I think, for me, that's the toughest bit of the menopause. So many of us women are incredibly strong when it comes to dealing with physical complaints – all the things like dry skin, dry eyes, dry mouth, or even dry vaginas. We can be resourceful and try to help ourselves, although I do hope that the beginning part of this book will help you to find really good ways of dealing with all of those symptoms.

But the one that really tears us apart is behaviour. When we turn into somebody we don't even recognise.

When we behave in a way that we abhor, that we are so ashamed of, and that can wreck careers and marriages and confuse people we care about who have got no idea what's going on and what's happened to the person that they knew and loved.

It has a catastrophic effect on everybody. It also has a really catastrophic effect in the workplace. Imagine the impact on the economy of losing all of these amazing women who are at the top of their game? We get to our forties and fifties, with all that experience, and we all start behaving in such a way that makes it almost untenable for us to stay in our jobs. Either we leave, or we are got rid of.

It's really, really hard, and anybody who is going through this, who is suffering themselves or struggling with their loved ones, and they hate themselves because they are literally powerless to do anything about it: I hear you. We hear you. We are all in this together.

We're going to hear the experiences of working women in this section, and their partners, and we're going to talk it all through.

'This is not me.' — Rachael

For many women, menopause is akin to driving a 10-tonne steamroller through every meaningful relationship, as Rachael's story shows:

*I'm forty and now on the second
different dosage and third type of HRT.
I'm still struggling. I wake up every day
more tired than I went to bed, my hair
is falling out, my skin is all scaly, I've got
spots all over my chin, my knees ache,
I'm always walking into things and it
takes ages for the bruises to fade.*

*My fifteen-year-old daughter went to
live with her dad because of my mood
swings and I've had so many rows
with my husband and his kids (my
stepchildren) over the years. But they
don't understand what I'm going
through, I can't explain it, I speak
but they don't seem to hear me.*

*About a year ago my husband and
I were at each other's throats all the
time. His kids used to hate coming
to ours because of the friction, the
atmosphere. They were scared to
breathe in case they woke the beast.
This has gone on for about two years,
and it does settle for a while with new
HRT, but I seem to become immune
eventually and the rollercoaster of
emotions starts again.*

*After being made redundant from my
last two jobs (the first of which I had
problems at because of my mood
swings), I've just failed my probation at
a new job because of the brain fog, the
lack of concentration and focus. I'm
worried that I now won't be able to
work as I can't seem to grasp new skills.*

*Sometimes I wonder where I went.
Who is this woman who struggles with
everything every day? This is not me.
I don't want to suffer anymore; I want a
resolution and to have energy and to
feel normal and to be me again.*

Rachael's story is heartbreaking.
Rachael, if you are reading this,
I would definitely ask for an appointment
with a menopause specialist. I know
sometimes these can be months away,
but I would persevere with trying to
find some kind of treatment that can
help you, because no one can carry on
shouldering the burden that you are.
Lots of love to you, Rachael.

I'm wondering if many of you are
recognising anything of yourselves
in Rachael's story – I know that the
menopause can really, really cause
enormous problems in all relationships.

In this chapter I just want to give some
pointers, because I know that I can't
wave a magic wand and suddenly make
it all better, but I do know that HRT
was a miraculous help for me.

It might be a bumpy ride, but it doesn't
necessarily have to be a disaster movie.
Relationships can be very difficult, but
communication, talking, sharing and
support from those who know you best
and love you the most is going to help
you through.

The best way to menopause-proof relationships and preserve your own sanity?

Start talking and KEEP TALKING

Probably the best time to try to talk to your friends, partners – even teenage children – and colleagues in your workplace is possibly not when you are in the throes of a hot flush or a flash of rage, or any other kind of debilitating symptom.

The best thing that you can do is wait until you are feeling relatively normal, sit people down and say, 'Look, I need to talk to you about what's going on, I'm really struggling.' Be as honest as you can. Let them in.

If you are really not coping, make that appointment to see a doctor. Go back to the previous chapter in this book; it will outline the things that you need to say to them – the things that you need to let them know – and talk about what treatment might be right for you.

If you are on some kind of a treatment but it just isn't working, it's not even touching the sides, make sure you go back and talk about that dosage, and again when they've tried a bigger dosage, then maybe a bigger dosage still. GPs, understandably, do start you off very low; they don't want to put you on a really high dosage straight away. Just remember, most people start on 25 microgram patches, and I'm on 100!

So know that there are places you can go in terms of dosage, but don't try to hide it from your partners or your friends – or even your kids, if you have them. These people love you and they are rooting for you, and they all want you to feel better.

WHY IT'S TIME TO EDUCATE

Often women say that when they try to explain it to people, they just don't understand. Sometimes if you are explaining it in terms of yourself, they might not fully comprehend the medical side of it, or the fact that it's not just happening to you, but that these are symptoms that happen to six hundred and sixty million other women around the world, and you just need a little help and support from them to get you through this.

In the days of the caveman, we used to look at paintings on the wall to inform ourselves, but nowadays you can find lots of information in a book like this, or you could go onto some of the amazing WhatsApp or Facebook groups. However you do it, you can share your story, but you can also take other people's stories and share them with your friends and family, so they can understand that it's not just you, this is a thing. Menopause is a thing, and something that makes life very difficult.

If you're finding it hard to put how you're feeling into words, maybe sit them down and give them something to read, or to watch or listen to.

So, things like:

→ This book (obvs).

→ *Sex, Myths and the Menopause* and *Sex, Mind and the Menopause* documentaries – they've got me in them! What more can you ask for?! They are a great introduction for partners in particular; they are only an hour each and cover everything we need to know in a non-judgemental way – symptoms, the myths and the facts.

→ Dr Naomi's Instagram – @drmenopausecare for all things perimenopause and menopause – symptoms, treatments. She also runs a Midweek Menopause Madness series with Lisa Snowdon @lisa_snowdon.

→ Gabby Logan's *The Mid•Point* podcast – guests talk about their midlife challenges and it has advice on everything from sleep to nutrition to hormones.

→ *Postcards from Midlife*: this podcast is literally me! In this, journalists Lorraine Candy and Trish Halpin are on a mission to help women make the most of their magnificent midlife.

CAN'T STAND THE SIGHT OF YOUR PARTNER?

People often compare menopause to the world's worst PMS. You know, that time of the month where, for one week, you just hate everything and everyone. And sometimes I think – well, I particularly felt this. Being menopausal can be a very, very lonely place; you can start feeling like you are the only person in the world that feels this way, and that no one understands what you're going through.

But if you're in a relationship, that person has loved you for years – and sometimes decades, right? We're in our forties and fifties, most of us, by the time this hits, and if they've loved you for decades then they're going to be there for you now.

I mean, let's just put the shoe on the other foot. Imagine how they're feeling – that sense of helplessness and being shut out when you can see the person you love is obviously in pain. A bit like when you give birth, and your partner is right there next to you in the birthing pool or labour suite, and they're holding your hand and they're trying to say the right things, but you're the life force at that moment, and they feel utterly helpless. They don't know what to do or what to say, and whatever they say it seems like the wrong thing.

Menopause is very similar – that feeling of *I don't know what to do, I don't know how to help.* Just like in giving birth, I think, it's really helpful if you say, '*This* is what I need you to do.'

'We blamed her menopause symptoms on malaria tablets.' — Peter

We're going to stop and look at it from another perspective for a second. Peter shared his story about what it was like seeing his wife struggling:

The first time I noticed a change in my forty-two-year-old wife was on holiday in Goa. We sat down for a meal and she burst into tears. 'I just want to go home,' she said. We put it down to the malaria tablets, as we were both experiencing side-effects. I wrapped my arms around her and said it will be ok, it's just the tablets.

Once we got home, though, I noticed her moods had changed. She was always normally in a good mood, but this wasn't the case now. She was angry and intolerant. The day she started screaming at me and chased me with a baseball bat we knew something was definitely wrong.

Peter, thank you so much for sharing your story with us – it is so important that we all get to see the other side of what it's like to live with someone who is seriously suffering with awful menopause symptoms.

Just to let you all know, thankfully there was a happy end to this story: Peter's wife went to see her GP and started HRT. It just reinforces the need to seek medical help.

Another issue you might be faced with is your partner wanting to take charge and 'fix' you. 'I know what to do,' they might say. 'This is what will take it away' – just do this, this, this and this, and bam – job done.

Except we know menopause just isn't like that. It's not that simple. And that can be hard for someone you love to get their head around, the fact that, as much as they want to, they can't just swoop in and make your problems disappear.

Ultimately, they end up feeling more useless, powerless and rejected than they did before. That's why you must keep on communicating, even in those moments when the mere sound of their voice feels like nails down a blackboard, or they've said the wrong thing *again*.

Of course we deserve sympathy by the bloody bucketload, but as ridiculous as it sounds, they deserve some of your sympathy, too.

If they offer help or want to know what's wrong, try to see it as coming from a good place. The keepers out there will want to listen, want to learn and want to see you better.

'It's easy to forget that menopause is hard for partners, too.' — Janine

Janine, another absolute warrior who shared her story of menopause at twenty-eight due to cancer treatment, summed it up this way:

Our partners really do go through it with us. But because they don't truly understand our feelings and the change to our bodies, it's easy to forget that it's hard for them, too. It was only on reflection later that I could see the change in his life and that his wife had changed forever.

Preach, Janine, I couldn't agree more.

A WORD TO ALL THE PARTNERS OUT THERE

Menopause can be a really lonely time for you, too, and it can be confusing to know what to do or say to your partner.

My top piece of advice for all the partners? Ask, don't assume.

The best way you can offer support is by asking 'what can I do to help?'. Find out what is the most useful, supportive thing you can do: do they want you to be their wingman at the doctor's, do they want to offload some admin they really can't face right now, do they want to be spoiled with a night away, or is it that they really, really just want a big old cuddle? You need to talk openly, honestly and often.

. . . .

'We burned a thousand joss sticks, tied ourselves in yoga knots, ran till we needed new trainers ... but still menopause seemed to be winning.' — Carl

Carl shared his story from a partner's perspective, and his words show just how tough it can be for the other halves. BUT the couple persevered, they got the care his partner needed, and things are on the up – and they could be for you, too.

I've been with my beautiful partner now for six years. When we got together, she was a happy, confident strong woman, but as time went on she started to change her outlook on life and found things difficult to deal with.

I tried to talk and listen to help her, but at the start neither of us could make sense of it. As time went on, we realised it was probably the menopause, so now all we had to do was beat this thing. EASY, right?

So we burned a thousand joss sticks, tied ourselves in yoga knots, I massaged till my fingers bled, ran till we needed new trainers, and ate so healthy we should live to be a thousand. But still it seemed to be winning.

Ok, plan two, let's get some professional medical help. Again, easy, right?

NOPE, wrong. You're depressed, they said, you have anxiety, you're stressed, take this pill, this will help. Your bloods are fine, it's not the menopause, you're too young. So that was three years and I couldn't see her suffer any more, so I said let's go private, let's see somebody that deals with this. To see a specialist your doctor has to refer you. Ok, appointment booked, time to sort this out. I watched her go into the clinic, thinking to myself all I wanted was for this doctor to say 'you're right', so at least we would know once and for all.

A six-month prescription and my girl has a look of relief. She's three months in now and although there are still some days that aren't perfect, the change is amazing. She feels like herself again and we have hope.

I will always remember what she said after her first day of treatment: 'I feel like I'm a teenager again' – those were the kind of words I dreamed of hearing.

Never give up. XXX

Oh my goodness, Carl, I am actually crying while I write this. The way you stuck by your partner and love-bombed her through what was a very difficult time, and then supported her and helped her get what she needed to try to become herself again is extremely moving. It's really lovely, and I'm so pleased that she's back to 'I feel like I'm a teenager again'. And you're absolutely right, Carl: never give up. Just keep battling on.

But, I think, very importantly what Carl has said here is showing us that sometimes it's so frightening when you're in it that you don't know how to get through it, and sometimes it takes the love of someone you really care about to carry you through the really tough bits. And the really tough bits are trying to get help, trying to get support from doctors or menopause specialists; the kind of medical help that you need. Sometimes you don't feel like you have a voice, and sometimes you need somebody with a voice to go along with you. So, bravo, Carl, I salute you.

THE RAGE AND HOW
TO DEAL WITH IT

The rage you can get with menopause when your hormones are out of whack can be a very scary place to be. You feel like you are about to flip a gasket, but at the same time you have no *fucking idea* why you are feeling like this.

Let me give you an example. When you are a parent, there are always those must-do tasks that feel never-ending. Now, I am by no means a screaming, shouty mum, but getting the kids out of the house in the morning is one of those real pressure points.

When my kids were very young, I used to set my alarm to get up just twenty minutes earlier than everyone else in the house. It was my time to get organised and take a breath. It was enough to make me feel like I wasn't starting the day on the back foot. Only twenty minutes, but it revolutionised the whole process of getting out of the door on time and in one piece. If you've got pre-school or school-age children and you aren't doing this, trust me, try it tomorrow. It really, really works.

But with perimenopause all that careful organisation and zen-like calm went out the window. The school run went from a finely tuned exercise of washed, dressed

and fed kids worthy of the Von Trapp family straight back to being the most stressful thing EVER. I morphed into this stressy, frantic mum.

And when the kids didn't move as quickly as I thought they should it felt like this huge tsunami of stress was building and building inside me, ready to spill over.

The rage was a very alien emotion for me. It wasn't the way that I would usually express my feelings, and I found it frightening and baffling. I just didn't get it. It had been a faff to get out of the door in the morning, but I had it sorted for so long ... so what was different now?

Suddenly I started taking it all very personally. Were the kids dawdling because they could see I was stressed? Was this just to push my buttons?

I would feel these flashes of irrational anger, but most of the time I kept a lid on it. I couldn't understand how I'd been coping with this for years and years and all of a sudden I just couldn't. It's a bit like if you have PMS; you never know when it will strike, what the trigger will be and how hard the emotions will hit you.

Once or twice I did lose it. And I felt AWFUL. I just broke down before starting the school run, apologising to my kids. The words came tumbling out in between sobs. 'I'm sorry, I don't know where that came from, it's not you, it's me. I'm not upset with you.'

HOW TO TALK TO YOUR KIDS ABOUT MENOPAUSE

For most of us who have children, when menopause hits your children will be at the point of being slightly older, and then you might have both teenage and menopause hormones under one roof.

I'd say that from the age of about eight or nine a child is old enough to be told in simple terms why Mummy feels like she's losing the plot sometimes. Children notice things, they hear things. They will more than likely have already clocked that something is up. You need to give them the credit that they will be able to understand, but you have to pitch the information in the right way.

As tempting as it is to try to belittle an issue or pretend it doesn't exist, it's always better to be honest. Rather than brushing your feelings under the carpet, get down to their level and explain in an age-appropriate way what's happening.

I remember those few times when I broke down on the school run. I was so worried about what the kids were thinking. Mummy's crying, that usually means something bad has happened. So I talked it through with them. I explained to them that it wasn't their fault, that I was crying because I was upset with myself, not with them.

'Something's going on in Mummy's body that makes her feel a bit all over the place,' I said. 'Sometimes I find it quite hard to control those feelings but I'm taking medication that is starting to level things out and make me feel a lot more human.'

TELL YOUR KIDS THEY CAN ASK YOU ANYTHING

From a really early age, I've made a point of telling my children they can ask me about anything. Birds, bees, periods –

anything. And the same should go for your menopause, too.

If you find it hard to verbalise it, keep a menopause diary and write it down. It doesn't have to be some massive book, it could just be 'today this happened, and this is how I felt about it'. It gives them a window into how you are feeling, why you might act the way you do sometimes, so they aren't left in the dark.

If you have grown-up kids you might need to have the menopause chat with them. They might not be as reliant on you if they've fled the nest, but you are still their mum.

Lend them a copy of this book. If you need their support and understanding, then you have to give them the tools so they are informed.

NEVER SAY SOMETHING YOU DON'T MEAN

As hard as it might be when you are in the heat of the moment, this is one really important rule to try to hold on to. Even if you are in the absolute depths of your darkest rage, never, ever say anything you don't *mean*.

Cher had it right. Words are like weapons, they wound sometimes.

There are some things that you can never unhear. What might be a momentary flip out for you during

a cross exchange of words or a full-on row could be a sentence that will be remembered by your kids, your other half, or your friends for the rest of their lives. And those few words can irreversibly change relationships.

IF YOU DO SAY SOMETHING YOU REGRET, REMEMBER, YOU ARE <u>NOT</u> THE WORST PERSON IN THE WORLD

If you do momentarily flip out and say something awful, stop, take a long, deep breath, own it and apologise. I'm not talking about a 'sorry you feel that way' or 'I'm sorry BUT...' type of apology, I mean a real heartfelt apology – it might not fix things right away, but it can go a long way.

KEEP YOUR FRIENDS CLOSE AND YOUR MENOPAUSING FRIENDS CLOSER

I can't stress this enough; if you don't already, you HAVE to start talking to your mates about menopause.

Quite often you find friends who aren't as menopause-savvy as you will be sitting there on their own wondering what on earth is going on inside their bodies. Do you want them to feel lost, lonely and clueless? No, of course you don't. You want the best for them, for them to be happy and thriving. So, get talking and start giving them some advice and some hope.

When it comes to menopause, there is no such thing as TMI. Bums, boobs, sex, sweats: next time you are out with your friends, talk about your mood swings, your brain fog, your hormones, your HRT patches, sprays and gels. Normalise this world for your friends, and for you, too.

You might find there comes a mic-drop moment when someone will say 'oh my God, I feel like that too' and you can tell them all about what you've learned.

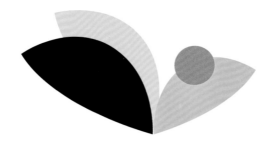

660 million women are heading for menopause worldwide and half are in the workforce.[1]

900,000 UK women have left their jobs because of menopause symptoms.[2]

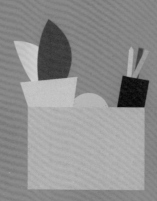

NAVIGATING WORKPLACE RELATIONSHIPS

When I was at home with my family, I felt I could cry and feel frustrated and let the emotion out, but at work it was a different story; I bottled it all up.

When I was struggling to find my words because my brain was full of fog, or I was feeling weepy, I would just try to hide it. And when I found myself unable to read the autocue I would think to myself, *that's it. I'm done. I can't do live TV anymore.* It felt completely overwhelming.

And I kept those feelings to myself, which was the absolute worst thing to do. If an outburst happens or brain fog descends while you are at work, it can definitely feel more embarrassing and scarier than if it happens at home or in the company of friends. And when you are frightened, you get defensive. This is the worst feeling in the world. (God, even the thought of anyone feeling like this makes me want to cuddle people.)

Your friends and family know the real you. At work, people will often only know the one side of you: that professional, I've-got-it-under-total-control work mode, so when you do

have an outburst, it can feel like you are losing control.

This is why I think so many women leave their jobs at this point. The demands and expectations are so high, so if you have a moment when you crumble or fall, it's not understood or looked on with empathy, but 'oh God, what's up with *her?*' 'Hot flushes? Oh, *here we go."*

A 2021 survey found that one in five menopausal women passed on the chance to go for a promotion that they would have otherwise considered, nineteen per cent reduced their hours and twelve per cent resigned.[3] Think how much this is worth to the economy alone. Think of all that knowledge, experience and power leaving the workplace because women in their fifties can't cope any more.

So many of you who shared your stories talked about how menopause was affecting your work – from fatigue to brain fog and everything in between – and here I want to share two stories with two very different outcomes for women's careers.

---

[1] www.news-medical.net/health/Menopause-and-the-Workplace.aspx (29.04.2022)

[2] Women and Equalities Committee Commons Select Committee, 'Women Menopause and the workplace Inquiry' https://committees.parliament.uk/work/1416/menopause-and-the-workplace/

[3] Balance (2021), 'Menopause symptoms are killing women's careers, major survey reveals', https://www. balance-menopause.com/news/menopause-symptoms-are-killing-womens-careers-major-survey-reveals/

'I quit the job I loved.' — Alison

First up, Alison, for whom it all got too much and she felt left with no other option than to walk away from her job.

In 2016 I quit my job as a police officer. I had been off work being treated for anxiety and depression but I never really felt like that was accurate. I took the decision to leave my career behind due to crippling brain fog. I couldn't find the correct words, I found making decisions hard and couldn't even remember the definitions relating to law that I knew so well and were vital for me to do my job properly. I resigned and no one asked any questions as to what could have been the cause of this rapid decline in my whole character.

I wanted to slip away unnoticed and I lived like a hermit for years. I started HRT nine months ago and can now see I was perimenopausal all along.

It's cost me so much, but I'm now a self-employed mosaic artist and have moved to the coast and use cold-water swimming as part of my therapy. If only one of the doctors had picked up on this five years ago... I'm sure if there had been the information I've found through Davina back then, things could've been different.

I just feel sad it cost me so much to get to this point. I miss helping people. That was what I was good at and I'll never get that back. Hopefully, raising awareness now means other women will be able to remain in their chosen careers and not go through what I have.

Alison, having read your story I find it totally heartbreaking because, as a nation, we have also clearly lost a really boss police officer, and I'm so sad about that. But I hope you are enjoying your mosaics – that sounds amazing – and I'm so pleased that you are feeling better now.

· · · · · · · ·

'I wear my HRT patch with pride and talk openly at work.' — Claire

Claire thought she was losing her mind as perimenopause entered her life, but with the support of her boss, family and

a well-informed GP, she managed to keep everything together when she thought it was all falling apart.

I knew at forty-seven it was likely I was perimenopausal but I just got on with feeling tired and forgetting things, but my bouts of rage were becoming increasingly worrying. Some days the way my family walked into a room would annoy me, I mean really annoy me, like I hated them.

At work, I became a prolific note-taker and list-maker in case I forgot things. Then one day I was sat in a client meeting with my boss and I remember thinking, 'What are everyone's names?' 'What is this meeting about?' I couldn't remember.

I managed to bluff my way through the meeting then headed to the train station. It was only when I got there I realised I had no idea where I lived. I stood for twenty minutes looking at the departure screens with tears rolling down my face. I thought I had dementia.

Eventually I found a train ticket in my purse, saw where I lived and got home. I drove to work the next day (using sat nav as I couldn't remember the way) and all I could think of was going into a home for people with dementia and how my children would cope.

As soon as I got to work, I was asked to go to my boss's office – I genuinely thought I was about to be sacked. I knew I hadn't been firing on all cylinders for weeks. He said he was worried about my work recently and obviously had picked up on the meeting the day before.

Then I broke down and told him I thought I had dementia. He was amazing and immediately his attitude was, 'What do we need to do to help you?'.

That night I filled out the online GP form with my husband's help, in tears. Within twenty-four hours my doctor called and reassured me I was highly likely menopausal and should try HRT – luckily she had had some training and told me how safe it was.

Now, five months on, I realise I don't have dementia and I love my family again!

I wear my patch with pride and talk openly at work. If I am having a tough day or if I'm angry at the world I let my colleagues know that 'dark Claire' is in the room so they can watch out and support me. My journey continues but I no longer feel alone.

I nearly lost my job. Could it also have cost me my sanity and my marriage if I hadn't had a good GP? Probably...

This is a great success story, Claire, because I felt exactly the same. I thought I had dementia – I was genuinely terrified. But I think it's fantastic that you got your husband's help, you filled out an online GP form and that your doctor called and diagnosed you as perimenopausal, AND got you on HRT. I mean, what a success right there! Well done for talking openly at work; you're going to help many more people and you are definitely not alone.

But thank you so much for sharing that, because it's important to hear positive stories, too. And I agree with you: God bless your GP! And well done boss!

Alison ended up walking out on a job that she loved and was good at because the right questions weren't asked. Not even when she handed in her notice. That makes me so mad.

In contrast, even though Claire was having a shitty time, her boss just got it. He picked up that something was wrong, sat her down for a one-to-one chat and asked what do we need to do to help you?

It is such a simple question, but one that is so important. Wrapped up in that was empathy, understanding and a recognition that it was up to the company to help Claire, not leave her to tough it out all alone. This is the reaction every woman should be getting from her employer.

Women don't want a fancy menopause workplace charter or people coming and sticking fans on everyone's desks (can you imagine all that paper flying through the air if they all got turned on at once?). They just want understanding, plain and simple.

Menopause doesn't have to be a 'thing'. We just need to normalise it. Talk about it. If you feel embarrassed to talk to your boss or your teammates, don't.

It sounds like a cliché but with age comes great experience. By the time of menopause you might be twenty or thirty years into a career. You've seen everything. You know everything. You are indispensable and, frankly, your employer would be mad not to do everything they can to keep you happy, thriving and kicking ass on their payroll.

You have real value. You ARE worth it. So be upfront about your menopause and the support you need – and here are some tips you can try today.

TALK TO YOUR COLLEAGUES

Don't do what I did and try to hide from the people you work with. If your brain feels like it has turned to mush and you can't remember the name of the person who you've sat next to at work for the past five years, don't feel mortified or try to style it out, tell them 'it's menopause – sometimes I forget names and dates'.

Or the next time a hot flush descends and it feels like the office or shop floor has turned into a fiery pit and you want to run away and hide under a pile of photocopier paper, don't. Stand your ground, face down any funny looks and normalise it.

Tell them: 'It's a hot flush. I'm menopausal. It happens. I'm going to head outside, cool down and come back.'

CAN'T TALK TO YOUR BOSS IN PERSON? HERE'S WHAT TO PUT IN A LETTER

→ Talking is always a good first option, but if you prefer to get your thoughts down on paper, or want it as backup, write a letter to your boss.

→ Be honest. Tell them, 'This is how I have been feeling and this is how it has affected my work'. Let them know your symptoms and describe how this has impacted you – is it brain fog? Hot flushes? What's going on?

→ Be proactive. Show you are trying to positively do something about your symptoms and tell them the steps you have already taken. Have you been to the doctor, are you taking HRT?

→ Be confident. Don't be afraid to ask for the help you need. This is a chance to change things. Would setting up a support group help you? Do you need some changes to the structure of your working day?

→ Be positive. Try to end the letter on an upbeat note. You want to be the best you can be at work, but to get back to where you should be you need some support and understanding.

WE NEED MENOPAUSING WARRIORS IN THE WORKPLACE

Ask about setting up a weekly menopause support group in a space where you can sit and share your experiences. Whether it's a weekly or a monthly thing, block it out in everyone's diaries and silence the phones so that everyone who wants to has the chance to attend.

These groups MUST include men. Men are our colleagues, our friends and our partners. The benefits of a group like that go beyond the walls of an office or workplace. You might have colleagues who have partners at home going through menopause and they have no idea how best to support them. They could really learn from listening and talking to other women about what they are going through, then they can support their partners, their sisters or their mums in the best way possible. Henpicked is a brilliant resource for menopause in the workplace training.

WORK FOR A BIG COMPANY? LOBBY FOR YOUR OWN MENOPAUSE CLINIC

We know the NHS is ridiculously over-stretched and access to specialist menopause clinics is a real postcode lottery. There are just under a hundred NHS menopause clinics in the UK,[4] which sounds like a lot on paper, but

---

[4] British Menopause Society, 'Find your nearest BMS menopause specialist', www.thebms.org.uk/find-a-menopause-specialist/?fbclid=IwAR3erCKWfLI8m-tX3BitMsCP4pbZpUyc2n-qvZDo9w6Mf1VgWMH8vIxoCnE

for something that half the population will go through, and thousands upon thousands of these women will need specialist support for, it really isn't. And if you do get a referral, there are places in Australia, the US and across the UK where women have to travel hundreds of miles for a face-to-face appointment. To put that into perspective, there are just twelve such clinics for the whole of Scotland, and only one in Northern Ireland.

Our health and our happiness is at stake here and we just can't afford to sit around and wait. This is an area where big business really needs to up its game; large corporations need to provide menopause clinics, and they need to create spaces for women to get help, support and advice. If not, the consequences will be women leaving their jobs because they can't cope, or losing their jobs because their menopause symptoms are being mistaken for under-performance.

NEED TO POINT YOUR BOSS IN THE RIGHT DIRECTION? SOME SOURCES OF INFO TO GET YOU STARTED

→ The **Chartered Institute of Personnel and Development** has guidance for managers on menopause in the workplace (www.cipd.co.uk)

→ **Women's Health Concern**, part of the British Menopause Society, has online resources on menopause and work (www.womens-health-concern.org)

→ The **Society of Occupational Medicine**, part of the Royal College of Physicians, has guidance on menopause and the workplace (www.som.org.uk)

AND IF THINGS DON'T IMPROVE: IS IT REALLY THE RIGHT JOB FOR YOU?

You've been to the GP about your symptoms, your boss has been brilliant and you've made a few changes at work for the better. But there's still a little voice in your head telling you this job isn't quite right.

And do you know what? That's ok. Let's not shy away from re-branding ourselves. Menopause is a time of change, and it can be a real time of clarity, too. Is there a career path you've always daydreamed about that you feel ready to try? Is now the time to go and change jobs and get out there and do something super-rewarding?

In some cases, leaving might be the best option. Speak to former colleagues who have moved on, or friends or families who have switched careers.

And if you want to feel inspired to make the switch, read on...

'I walked out on a 30-year career – now I run my own business.' — Sarah

For Sarah, menopause meant reinventing herself and starting again using skills she had learned over a thirty-year career, but also finding real satisfaction in her new role.

I'd been working as an NHS nurse for thirty years. I was a senior community nurse working with vulnerable children and safeguarding. I'd raised a family of four. My identity was as a mum and a nurse. I hit forty-eight and everything changed.

I began to feel anxious at work, I was suffering from headaches, irritable bowel syndrome symptoms, raised blood pressure, brain fog and a lack of confidence. Following what I can only describe as a panic attack at work, I walked out and never went back!

I sat on my sofa for six months staring at the walls with my daughter trying to encourage me with 'mindful colouring' and piano lessons, and my son talking to me as if I was hard of hearing! They had never seen their mum like this.

I had counselling and was told I was totally burnt out and was encouraged not to return to nursing. I had lost my identity; if I wasn't a nurse then what was I? What could I do?

I had to reinvent myself. Fast-forward five years and I am now running my own thriving business, delivering paediatric first aid courses across Sussex. I teach new and expectant parents, childcare providers and children in schools and I love it! I'm loving the flexibility of running my business and never thought it was possible. It's been a steep learning curve and I still help out my old nursing teams – I was involved in the Covid-19 vaccination programme.

I realise that what I went through five years ago was perimenopause and if I had had more knowledge of this and more support at work things might have been very different. But I have learnt so much about myself and the strength I've had to start my own business, become a social media queen and understand the importance of networking and meeting some amazing and inspiring women in business.

Thanks for sharing your story Sarah, I love hearing about women at this time in their lives starting their own businesses – it is so inspiring.

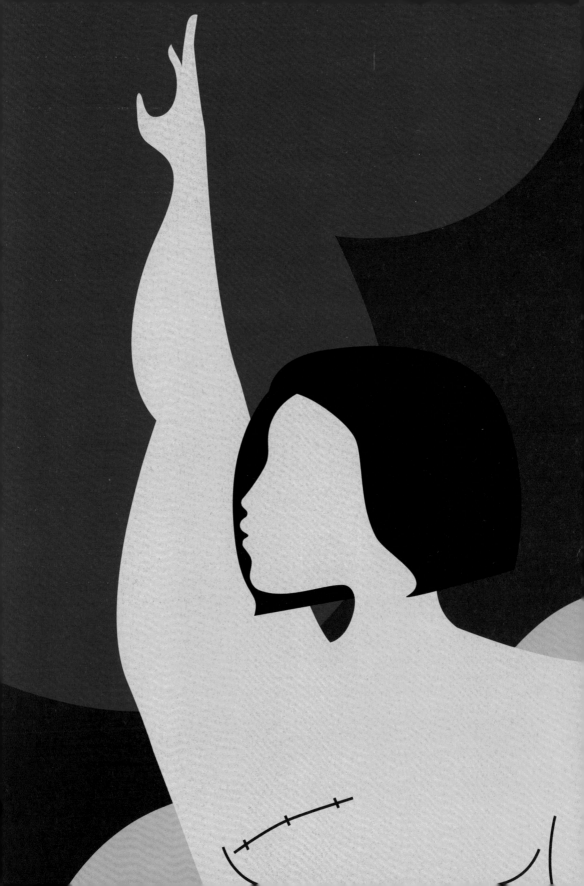

CHAPTER 11

DEALING WITH MENOPAUSE ALONGSIDE BREAST CANCER: ADVICE ABOUT HRT AND NON-HORMONAL TREATMENT OPTIONS

'Red nail varnish and my biker jacket ... come hell or high water you AIN'T taking those from me.'

'I would just love to be HEARD.'

When I read through your hundreds of stories, it was so clear that so many of you are coping with menopause alongside breast cancer. Some of you spoke about amazing care and support, but others were given mixed messages, or little or no information to go on, and just left to figure it out themselves.

In 2020 alone, 2.3 million women were diagnosed with breast cancer worldwide.[1] So in this chapter, Dr Naomi is going to give you the tools to manage menopause, the questions you can ask to get the information you need, as well as treatment options. For those of you who are unable, or don't want to take HRT, we have a run down of other non-hormonal treatments and therapies that can help.

DR NAOMI: TREATMENT OPTIONS IF YOU HAVE A HISTORY OF CANCER

Women with cancer, especially with a history of breast cancer, can often feel overlooked when it comes to menopause care. I find that women who have or have had breast cancer feel very left out of the menopause conversation and that really needs to change.

I'VE HAD BREAST CANCER. CAN I TAKE HRT?

The latest study confirms what we already thought was the case that oestrogen-only HRT does not increase the risk of breast cancer. Oestrogen plus micronised (body-identical) progesterone is also not associated with an increased risk of breast cancer. Oestrogen with synthetic progesterone is associated with a small increased risk of breast cancer.[2]

---

[1] World Health Organization (2021), 'Breast Cancer', https://www.who.int/news-room/fact-sheets/detail/breast-cancer

Not all breast cancers are the same. Some cancers have hormones receptors on them and some don't. If they have receptors they can grow under the influence of hormone. About seventy-five per cent of all breast cancers have receptors for oestrogen and are called oestrogen-receptor positive or ER positive (ER+) breast cancer. Officially, HRT should not be given to any woman with a history of breast cancer.[3] However, sometimes if a woman had breast cancer a very long time ago, or if it was very localised, it might be possible to take HRT under the guidance of a specialist. Also, if your cancer was not hormone receptor positive then it may be safer to give HRT but, again, this would usually be under the guidance of a specialist. When making the decision about starting HRT or using alternative therapies, I always discuss every woman's individual history and own wishes and weigh up the pros and cons of HRT with them.

WHAT ABOUT A FAMILY HISTORY OF BREAST CANCER?

Women with a family history of breast cancer are often told they can't take HRT, which in fact is often not the case. If you have a strong family history of breast cancer (for example, your mum or sister were diagnosed with breast cancer before the age of forty) you are more likely to develop breast cancer, but it is not thought that HRT will raise your overall risk. I would advise speaking to a specialist before deciding on whether to take HRT. If you have a family history of breast cancer, you can ask your doctor for a referral to a specialist family history clinic or a regional genetics centre to find out more.

'I'm jealous of women that can merrily neck their HRT.' — Darlaine

[2] Abenhaim et al. (2022), 'Menopausal Hormone Therapy Formulation and Breast Cancer Risk', American College of Obstetricians and Gynecologists

[3] Cancer Research UK (2020), 'Tests on Your Breast Cancer Cells', https://www.cancerresearchuk.org/about-cancer/breast-cancer/getting-diagnosed/tests-diagnose/hormone-receptor-testing-breast-cancer

Darlaine was diagnosed with invasive lobular breast cancer, a cancer that begins in the milk-producing glands in the breast, in 2016 when she was fifty-five.

Not really much of a menopause feeling at that point, odd low mood. Double mastectomy, followed six months later by having my ovaries removed, over that damn cliff, then plunging into menopause hell with only a pair of flippers to scramble back up with.

What kind of fuckery is this? I thought. It's made worse for me and others with hormone-positive breast cancer by the medication that I have to take to suppress oestrogen further. Grown a bloody goatee that you could moor a ship to, plucking takes the strength of Arnie. Nightmare joint pains, ankles and hips especially, I rise from a chair with the groans of that old aunt with the bingo wings that hang in folds as they push themselves up.

My skin and hair have lost their lustre, and I have a dried-up, withering vag.

I'm jealous of women that can merrily neck their HRT. A small offering of sanity is local oestrogen gel for my dried-up womanhood, and red nail varnish and my biker jacket. Come hell or high water, you ain't taking those from me.

Darlaine – Christ alive! I can't imagine what you've been through, and no one will **ever** take your red nail varnish and your biker jacket. So coming up we are going to go through all the possible things that could help you that aren't HRT. **Keep reading!**

THE ALTERNATIVES: NON-HORMONE TREATMENTS FOR MENOPAUSE

Menopause isn't always just about HRT. Some women can't or don't want to use HRT, and that is completely their choice. Being told you can't have HRT, or deciding it isn't for you, can leave women feeling lost. In particular, those with a history of breast cancer can feel very forgotten in menopause conversations.

You can revisit Chapter 6 for some specific advice on whether you can take HRT if you have a history of cancer or other health conditions. But if you are unable to, please be reassured that there are options available and, in Dr Naomi's experience, these can be effective at reducing symptoms.

Here are some of the medical options that you can discuss with a healthcare professional.

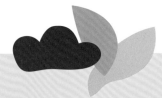

DR NAOMI: NON-HORMONAL TREATMENT OPTIONS

ANTIDEPRESSANTS (SSRIS AND SNRIS)

What can it help with? Low mood and anxiety, hot flushes and night sweats.

As we saw in Chapter 7 on menopause and mental health, antidepressants shouldn't be a first-line treatment for menopause-related low mood, but they might be an option for anxiety, low mood or hot flushes if you are unable or don't want to take HRT. They can be very effective but side-effects like nausea, dry mouth and low libido can occur.

Note: if you are taking tamoxifen, a medication that is used to treat oestrogen-receptor-positive breast cancer, you should not take the antidepressants paroxetine or fluoxetine as they can interact.

CLONIDINE

What can it help with? Hot flushes.

Clonidine is best known as a blood pressure medication, but it is also licensed for use for hot flushes and sweats. Side-effects include dizziness.

GABAPENTIN

What can it help with? Primarily hot flushes but it can help with sleep.

Gabapentin is a drug with many uses including epilepsy and nerve pain. It can reduce hot flushes in about half of patients,[4] and it can also help relieve pain and improve sleep. Results vary and side-effects can include drowsiness, dizziness and weight gain. It is a controlled drug, so there are strict rules over prescribing it.

OXYBUTYNIN

What can it help with? Hot flushes.

Oxybutynin is a drug that has been used to treat overactive bladder but has also been shown to help with hot flushes. It is non-hormonal so can be used in women with a history of breast cancer and is usually well tolerated but can cause dry mouth.[5]

NEUROKININ 3 RECEPTOR ANTAGONISTS

What can it help with? Hot flushes and sweats.

Neurokinin 3 receptor antagonists are an exciting development in treatment of menopausal flushes and sweats for women who cannot take hormones. Research has shown that oestrogen loss in menopause increases a hormone called neurokinin B. Neurokinin B stimulates neurokinin 3 receptors which in turn affect the temperature-controlling centre in the brain, so the pathway is overstimulated if oestrogen is low. If these receptors are blocked, the pathway can be suppressed, and symptoms reduced.[6]

VAGINAL MOISTURISERS AND LUBRICANTS

Vulvovaginal dryness can be a side-effect of menopause as well as some cancer treatments including breast cancer treatments. Vaginal moisturisers and lubricants can be particularly helpful as they are non-

---

[4] British Menopause Society 'Prescribable alternatives to HRT', https://thebms.org.uk/wp-content/uploads/2018/03/Prescribable-alternatives-to-HRT-01EE.pdf

[5] R.A. Leon-Ferre, P.J. Novotny, E.G Wolfe, et al, (2019), 'Oxybutynin vs placebo for hot flashes in women with or without breast cancer'

[6] British Menopause Society (2020), 'New non-hormonal treatment for hot flushes', https://thebms.org.uk/2020/07/new-non-hormonal-treatment-for-hot-flushes/

hormonal and risk free. I recommend looking for those which are pH and osmolality balanced – see Sam's chapter for more details. It is important not to forget that topical vaginal oestrogens do not carry the same risks of systemic HRT and can often be used in women with a history of breast cancer under the advice of their specialist.

OTHER THERAPIES

CBT is a psychological therapy recommended by NICE to alleviate low mood and anxiety, and it can improve hot flushes and sweats. It's advantages are it is medication free, so there are no side effects. It can, however, be time consuming and isn't always available on the NHS so can be expensive.[7]

Mindfulness and meditation can help with mood symptoms and promote more restful sleep.[8]

Acupuncture some women report very good results from acupuncture although this may be due to a high placebo effect.

Massage and reflexology also have some evidence of efficacy.[9]

DON'T FORGET LIFESTYLE MEASURES, TOO

Lifestyle plays an important part in menopause management. A well-balanced diet and reducing sugar and refined foods can improve symptoms. Alcohol and spicy foods cause the blood vessels to expand, known as vasodilation. This in turn makes you feel warmer and can trigger or exacerbate hot flushes. Caffeine perpetuates adrenaline and stimulates its release which can exacerbate anxiety and negatively impact sleep. The next chapter has lots of advice and tips on how a healthy lifestyle can help.

---

[7] 'Nonhormonal management of menopause-associated vasomotor symptoms: 2015 position statement of The North American Menopause Society', *Menopause*.

[8] D.S Oliveira, H. Hachul, H, V. Goto, S. Tufik, L.R Bittencourt (2012), 'Effect of therapeutic massage on insomnia and climacteric symptoms in postmenopausal women', Climacteric : the journal of the International Menopause Society.

[9] Z. Abedian, et al. (2015), 'The Effect of acupressure on sleep quality in menopausal women: a randomized control trial', Iranian Journal of Medical Sciences.

WHAT ABOUT HERBAL MEDICINES?

It's very common for women to try herbal medicines to ease symptoms, yet studies on efficacy are limited and the potency of preparations varies. The following has been compiled from the British Menopause Society recommendations and my own experience of prescribing.

Black Cohosh is a North American traditional herb that can help with hot flushes but isn't as effective as HRT. It can also interact with other medication and there are unknown risks regarding safety and liver toxicity.

Gamma-Linolenic Acid (GLA) is a fatty acid found in evening primrose oil and starflower oil. It has anti-inflammatory properties and can be helpful if you suffer from PMS-type symptoms like breast tenderness. Evidence is limited.

Ginseng and other Chinese herbal remedies have no evidence of efficacy although anecdotally some patients report that they help.

Isoflavones are a type of phytoestrogen, which is similar to the oestrogen produced in our bodies. Found in red clover, soy products and supplements, isoflavones have inconsistent results and show little value. They are not usually recommended for women with a history of breast cancer.

St John's Wort is a flowering plant that can help with hot flushes or night sweats and low mood. However, safety and reliability are a concern, and it has many drug interactions.

If you've had any kind of cancer diagnosis, past or present, it's worth talking to your oncologist, gynaecologist and menopause specialist, ideally together, as they will be able to work as a team to come up with the very best course of action for you. You deserve to receive the best treatment. Good luck.

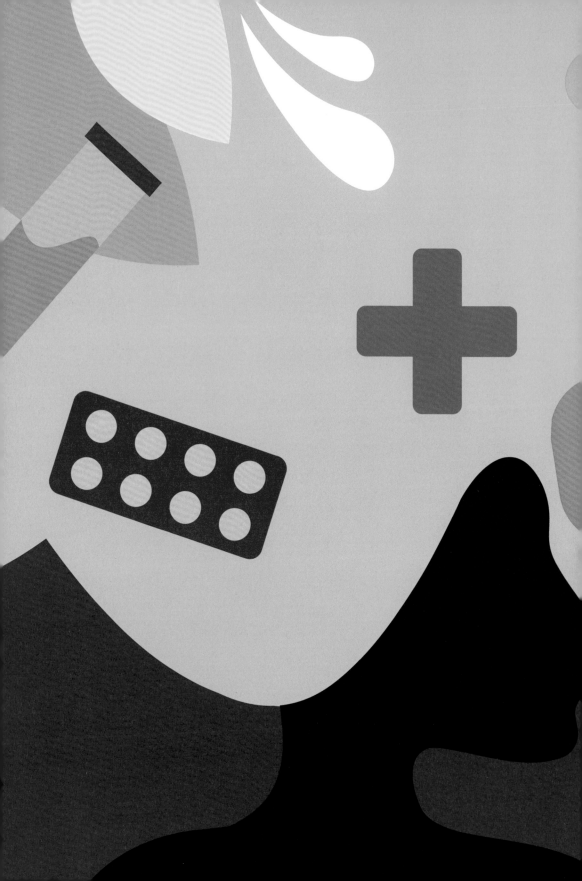

CHAPTER 12

DEALING WITH MENOPAUSE AND OTHER HEALTH CHALLENGES

● ● ● ● ● ● ● ● ● ●

One in ten women suffer from endometriosis.[1]

● ● ● ●

Three out of four will suffer from PMS.[2]

● ●

One in two of us will be diagnosed with cancer at some point in our lifetime.[3]

● ● ● ● ● ● ● ● ● ●

And every single one of us will go through menopause.

We aren't just statistics. We all deserve the right advice, support and care. From ovarian cancer to other conditions like endometriosis and thyroid issues, so many of you who shared your stories talked about your struggles with coping with menopause and managing other health problems at the same time.

[1] K.T Zondervan et al. (2020), 'Endometriosis', The New England Journal of Medicine.

[2] M. Steiner (2000), 'Premenstrual syndrome and premenstrual dysphoric disorder: guidelines for management', Journal of Psychiatry and Neuroscience.

[3] NHS.uk (2019) 'Overview: cancer', https://www.nhs.uk/conditions/cancer/

'Menopause after cancer treatment: what I say can be disregarded by women who have started menopause naturally.' — Janine

When she was in her teens and early twenties, Janine couldn't wait for her periods to end, because she hated the hassle and the pain they brought.

Now I feel so annoyed with myself and feel pretty stupid that I wished for menopause.

I started my menopause at age twenty-eight due to cancer treatment that caused my ovaries to fail. I started HRT a year later due to unbearable menopause symptoms. The night sweats, emotional instability, lack of sex drive and feeling like a crazy woman were not pleasant experiences.

The big moment when I asked for help was when I walked to work one day happy, and by the time I had taken my coat off I had started to cry. Not a little cry, a full-on sobbing, shoulder-shrugging cry. My colleagues must have thought something horrendous and traumatic had happened... I didn't have a clue what was happening.

After locking myself in a toilet for thirty minutes, I realised I couldn't stay there all day so I decided to brave it at my desk. Sobbing, I made my way to my desk and everyone was watching, so I decided the rational thing to do was tell everyone not to look at me and roll my chair over to the corner of the room. I just sat there until the tears stopped.

I have now been on HRT for eight years and see it as my lifeline. They say Red Bull gives you wings, well, HRT gives me life.

Although I try to speak about menopause, as I feel it's important, I can't help but feel disappointed when what I say is disregarded by another woman who has started menopause naturally. I look forward to the days when we can all talk about it without feeling awkward and can support each other at any stage of menopause.

Thank you for sharing, Janine. Cancer and HRT is such a complicated issue – we must keep talking and educating each other.

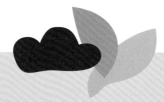

DR NAOMI: COPING WITH CANCER AND MENOPAUSE

A cancer diagnosis can be really tough, let alone being told your treatment may mean menopause earlier than you expected.

You may therefore be coping simultaneously with cancer treatment and menopause.

It's very common for women with any personal or family history of cancer to be told they can't have HRT under any circumstances. However, this may not always be the case, and it means some women who have severe symptoms and who could benefit from HRT are left to struggle on.

If you have a history of cancer, I'd recommend that you see someone with specialist knowledge to discuss your options. It is important that you have a discussion about your own personal circumstances and weigh up the risks and benefits. It is about teasing out what is the right thing in every single case.

If HRT is not suitable, there are alternatives which we covered in the previous chapter. These can help bring

relief from symptoms like hot flushes and vaginal and urinary symptoms. And don't forget to try lifestyle adjustments.

Cancer treatments that can put you into menopause are:

→ Surgery involving the ovaries.

→ Chemotherapy.

→ Radiotherapy to the pelvic area.

→ Hormone treatments.

Surgery to remove both ovaries will result in a permanent sudden surgical menopause, while for other treatments your menopause may be temporary or permanent. This will depend on the treatment and your age as the older you are the more likely it will be irreversible.

I have seen women whose lives have been turned upside down by having their ovaries removed without a full explanation of the ramifications of a surgical menopause. I've been told of women having been advised, 'We may as well remove them while we are in there', 'You won't even notice', and 'You've had your babies so you don't need them anymore.' It is often absolutely necessary to remove the ovaries but the consequences should not be downplayed.

Your ovaries are responsible for the vast majority of your oestrogen and a significant amount of testosterone production. When they are removed, for whatever reason, there will be an immediate surgical menopause. That immediacy means you are more likely to suffer more severe symptoms.

You have the right to expect a full discussion about the surgery and the side-effects.

What to ask your cancer specialist:

→ What will this treatment mean for me – will my menopause be temporary or permanent?

→ How will it affect my fertility?

→ What treatments can I have for menopause symptoms – and can you prescribe them today?

If you need more information, ask to be referred to a menopause specialist.

'Menopause is a lonely place for many women, myself included.' — Heather

Heather is going through surgical menopause at the age of thirty-three. In 2020, she was diagnosed with a rare form of cancer called leiomyosarcoma, following emergency surgery to remove a ruptured fibroid.

The cancer was found to be oestrogen-receptor-positive, so I chose to have my ovaries removed in the hope that it would reduce my risk of recurrence.

So I'm now going through surgical menopause, and it has been a struggle. I can't take HRT. The hot flushes are pretty awful, and I'm having to learn to live with this. It's particularly hard because I have a two-year-old son and I'm still trying to be active and do stuff with him, but it's difficult when I'm out and about and I get a hot flush and just start sweating profusely. I find it really embarrassing and awkward.

As well as the physical side-effects, menopause has had a real impact on my mental health. I have struggled with anxiety and low mood for a while, but the menopause (and a cancer diagnosis) have made it worse. I also find it difficult to concentrate and struggle with brain

fog, and I have difficulty remembering things. All of these things have been particularly difficult in relation to work. Trying to explain how I feel and how it's impacting me has been a real challenge, as it's hard to articulate these problems to people who haven't been through this themselves.

I reached a really low point where my mood was really suffering, but thankfully I have now started taking a type of antidepressant called escitalopram, and this seems to be helping. There is some evidence to show that this drug can help with hot flushes as well, but we'll have to wait and see if they improve.

Menopause is a lonely place for many women, myself included. I can't talk to my peers about what I'm experiencing because they're at such a different stage of life, many of them having babies, etc. It has been mentioned a couple of times that maybe I'll be able to take HRT in the future, but my cancer is so rare and there is so little evidence and knowledge about it that I don't know if I'll ever feel able to. At the same time, I am worried about the impact of early menopause on my long-term health, so I'm trying to keep myself as healthy as possible through diet and exercise, such as weight-bearing exercises. I'm also going to be having regular DEXA scans.

Thank you so much for your story, Heather. Sending so much love to you.

. . . .

'I'd love to feel heard and guided.' — Kris

For over fifteen years, Kris has suffered with endometriosis and PMDD (premenstrual dysphoric disorder), and describes living a life of pain and suicidal thoughts.

From the endometriosis, I would bleed heavily for seven to nine days. It caused a lot of discomfort; sex was extremely painful for days afterwards. I then got diagnosed with fibromyalgia [a long-term condition that causes pain all over the body] and altogether I felt my body was shutting down on me.

The PMDD had me feeling suicidal ten days before every period and would ease on the day of my period. I was just existing, not living. I felt I couldn't take any more and a hysterectomy seemed the only way out of suffering. Honestly, I felt great afterwards. I felt alive. I tried HRT but my PMDD came back, this scared me as I didn't want my life to go back to what I felt I'd finally been freed from. The fear of this never truly got understood by my doctors and they

suggested antidepressants would help. I knew this to not be true for myself so I don't take anything, but my body is calling out for what it's missing. I feel at a loss over what to do for the best... I would just love to be heard and guided to the correct input so my body can feel fulfilled.

Thank you so much for talking about PMDD, Kris. It's very important; not enough women talk about it, and it is not spoken about enough in the press or in magazines. And I'm pretty sure many women are suffering from PMDD and aren't even aware that they are. There are added complications to this, especially when it comes to taking things like hormones of any kind – because of the hormone fluctuations. So, thank you so much for sharing your story.

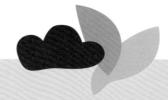

DR NAOMI: OTHER CONDITIONS AND MENOPAUSE

PMS AND PMDD

Both PMS and PMDD can worsen during perimenopause. Using HRT can help but finding the right dose and method of delivery, can be a challenge.

My advice is that if you have PMS or PMDD, make a point of bringing that into your initial conversation and ask to see a specialist.

Because you are sensitive to hormonal fluctuations, starting HRT can trigger PMS-type symptoms like anger, rage, tearfulness, breast tenderness and bloating. These can be addressed by altering the dosage or trying a different delivery method.

ENDOMETRIOSIS

About one in ten women of reproductive age in the UK suffer from endometriosis,[4] where tissue similar to the lining of the uterus begins growing in places elsewhere in the body. Whereas the lining of the uterus (known as the endometrium) builds up each month and then sheds during a period, the tissue elsewhere in the body has nowhere to go. This can lead to pain and scar tissue forming and symptoms such as:

→ Pelvic pain.

→ Period pain.

→ Pain during or after sex.

→ Bowel issues such as constipation and diarrhoea.

→ Urinary symptoms.

→ Difficulty getting pregnant – the prevalence of endometriosis in women with infertility can be as high as 30–50 per cent.[5]

→ Fatigue.

---

[4] P.A.W Rogers, et al. (2009). 'Priorities for endometriosis research: recommendations from an international consensus workshop', Reproductive Sciences, 16 (4), pp. 335-46. Doi.org/10.1177/1933719108330568

[5] L.J. Baker, P.M.S O'Brien, (2012), 'Premenstrual syndrome (PMS): a peri-menopausal perspective', Maturitas, 72 (2), pp. 121-5, doi.org/10.1016/j.maturitas.2012.03.007

While there is no cure, there are ways to manage the symptoms. These include pain relief, hormone treatment to slow endometrial tissue growth and prevent new deposits, and surgery.

When it comes to endometriosis and menopause, treatment can be quite complex, so I would always advise being referred to a menopause specialist.

HRT is an option. However, endometrial deposits outside of the uterus can be stimulated by the additional oestrogen. While this doesn't rule out HRT completely, you should see a specialist to discuss what is right for you.

In the majority of cases, women who have had their uterus removed will not need progesterone, but one exception is endometriosis as you can still have areas of endometrium in your body.[6]

Lifestyle changes (exercise and cutting out alcohol, sugar and coffee) can help.

The charity Endometriosis UK has some really helpful information on endometriosis and menopause, as well as a free helpline (www.endometriosis-uk.org).

THYROID CONDITIONS

Women are ten times more likely to suffer from thyroid disorders than men.[7]

There are two types:

→ Hypothyroidism, where the thyroid is underactive and doesn't produce enough thyroid hormones.

→ Hyperthyroidism, where the thyroid is overactive and produces too much of the thyroid hormones.

Both types of thyroid disorder can cause symptoms such as mood changes, metabolic and weight changes, tiredness and sensitivity to different temperatures. Symptoms can be similar to perimenopause.

As we saw earlier in the book, thyroid problems are more likely to occur in women with early menopause or POI and vice versa. In addition, declining oestrogen during perimenopause and menopause can also have an impact on thyroid hormone replacement requirements.

[6] H. Hamoda, N. Panay, H. Pedder, R. Arya R, M. Savvas, (2020) 'The British Menopause Society and Women's Health Concern 2020 recommendations on hormone replacement therapy in menopausal women, Post Reproductive Health, 26(4), pp.181-209. Doi.org//10.1177/2053369120957514

[7] British Thyroid Foundation (2021), 'Thyroid and menopause', www.btf-thyroid.org/thyroid-and-menopause

HAVE A THYROID DISORDER AND TAKING HRT? HERE'S WHAT YOU NEED TO KNOW

Having a thyroid disorder shouldn't be a barrier to taking HRT, but there is an interplay between the two that is poorly understood due to lack of research. Here are the key points to be aware of:

→ Thyroid hormone requirements can increase at perimenopause. HRT may reduce those requirements although data is lacking.

→ Although it is typically oral oestrogen replacement that affects thyroid hormone levels, it's worth asking your doctor to check your thyroid function (via a blood test) after you start taking HRT if you feel any of your thyroid symptoms returning.

MENOPAUSE AND HIV

Almost 100,000 people in the UK are living with HIV.[8] HIV and menopause is under-researched, but studies have shown that women living with HIV are more likely to go into menopause at an earlier age, especially if they have a low CD4 count (a white blood cell that destroys some bacteria and viruses).

A 2021 UK study of 836 women living with HIV found a third reported severe menopausal symptoms, but less than half had heard of HRT and less than one in ten used it. Just five per cent of women with urogenital symptoms had used topical oestrogen.[9]

The reasons are not clear but it is thought it could be due to HIV or the immune system's impact on the ovaries and their production of hormones that affect the experience of menopause.

HIV and some HIV treatment may (like menopause) increase the risk of developing osteoporosis.[10]

HRT can be taken with HIV treatment, but speak to your doctor to check if there are any interactions between HRT and the anti-HIV drugs you're on.

---

[8] National AIDS Trust (2021), 'HIV in the UK statistics', www.nat.org.uk/about-hiv/hiv-statistics

[9] H. Okhai et al. (2021), 'Menopausal status, age and management among women living with HIV in the UK', HIV Medicine, 22(9), pp. 834-42. Doi.org/10.1111/hiv.13138

[10] Terrence Higgins Trust (2021), 'Osteoporosis', www.tht.org.uk/hiv-and-sexual-health/living-hiv-long-term/osteoporosis

'I had a surgical menopause and have a thyroid disease – but I'm getting there.' — Sophie

Sophie had her ovaries removed after she was diagnosed with fibroids – she had three fibroids, the largest of which was ten centimetres in diameter.

Six weeks later I started oestrogen-only HRT and was prescribed 0.5mg/day of gel, gradually increased to 2mg as my symptoms were quite severe.

My situation was complicated by the fact that I was diagnosed with hypothyroidism towards the end of 2017 and subsequently Hashimoto's disease [an autoimmune disease where the immune system attacks the thyroid]. I now know that the thyroid and oestrogen interact with each other and have comparable symptoms, so I wasn't sure what was causing what.

I wasn't suffering from hot flushes but a sensation of heat, which would usually strike in the morning and late in the evening. I had terrible fatigue, trouble sleeping, loss of energy, irritability, anxiety and pain during intercourse and my libido was also on the floor. Again, it was difficult to assess whether this was the consequence of the menopause or the onset of the Hashimoto's disease.

In January 2021 I saw a menopause specialist; she just totally got everything

and understood exactly why I was feeling so bad. I had an oestradiol blood test that showed my oestrogen level was far too low and I wasn't absorbing the gel, so she switched me to transdermal patches. She also prescribed testosterone gel, which is something that had never been mentioned to me before.

I had a follow-up appointment with the same menopause doctor and she increased the oestrogen dose again, and a subsequent oestradiol blood test showed that my oestrogen is much better. I'm getting there!

Thank you for your story, Sophie. It just highlights the need for more menopause specialists, especially within the NHS. I'm so glad they could help you, and that your oestrogen levels are getting much better. High five!

What we can see from this chapter is that every single case and every single woman is an individual with very individual needs. It is worth doing your research by reading this book and arming yourself with the correct questions to ask your doctor. Knowledge is power.

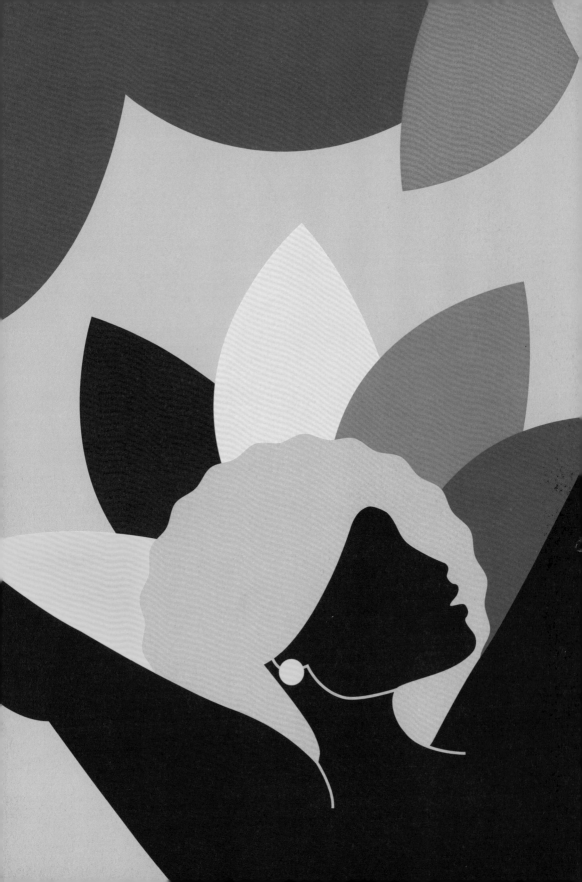

CHAPTER 13

I SEE YOU – AND YOU LOOK F***** GREAT: POSITIVE CHANGES DURING THE CHANGE

Getting back to your best during perimenopause and menopause needs more than just hormones and other medication. Exercise, eating right and just generally taking the time to look after number one are non-negotiables and need to be part of your menopause plan.

Don't know where to start? From exercises through to the vitamins and nutrients you can't afford to miss in your diet, I've got it covered. Plus I have some amazing tips from queen of skincare Caroline Hirons, make-up tips from Cheryl Phelps-Gardiner and haircare guru Michael Douglas on how to feel and look your best.

GET MOVING

Fitness was never really a thing for me during my childhood or in my teens. In my early twenties, my main workout was clubbing. Six hours of dancing was pretty good cardio! But when I hit my mid-twenties and stopped clubbing, quit smoking, quit alcohol and got clean, my weight ballooned.

I resolved to do something about it so I started working out. At first, I had no clue. I joined a gym, but it was a complete waste of time and money because I had no idea how any of the machines worked and was too embarrassed to ask. I just hung around in active wear trying to look cool, like I knew what I was doing.

Exercise really only clicked into place for me when I was pregnant with my second child, Tilly, and I met Jackie and Mark Wren through a local magazine.

Anybody who has done any of my workout DVDs will know Jackie and Mark, because they did the majority of my DVDs with me. They helped inspire me to love exercise; it really was down to them.

I wanted to look better and feel better, but I really just wanted to look after myself more so I could, in turn, look after the two kids that I had (and I was pretty sure I was going to have another one, if I was lucky).

Exercise has been a big part of my life ever since. And look, as I've got older my exercise routine has slightly changed. I may have slowed down a bit – I used to do a lot of HIIT and quite extreme cardio in my late thirties and forties. I've always exercised at least three or four times a week, but I used to really push myself back then, and I don't beast myself in that way anymore. I'm a bit calmer about it all.

I know what exercise I enjoy, I know what really works for my body rather that what I think I *should* be doing. That's a change in myself – I think as I've got older I understand myself a lot better and don't beat myself up about things.

But in those early days of perimenopause, it was like I'd run out of steam. Hot flushes, lack of sleep … I really lost the motivation to exercise, especially in the mornings. I mean, really, does anybody jump out of bed at six o'clock in the morning, screaming 'Yipeee!' about a dawn run or a HIIT workout that they're about to do? No, I don't think they do.

I did *know* that after a workout I would be glad I had done it, but when I was perimenopausal I just couldn't face it. I hadn't slept at night, I just felt SO unmotivated. And that actually frightened me because I'd always been so motivated about exercise up until that point.

When I started HRT that changed: the hot flushes and night sweats went, I felt more focused and my energy levels were back. Ok, so I still wasn't *completely* over the moon at the thought of getting up super-early to exercise, but I still did it. And after I worked out I'd be so chuffed that I did.

WHY YOU NEED TO EXERCISE DURING MENOPAUSE

Exercise is massively important at any time of our lives, but it really does come into its own during perimenopause and menopause. The crashing hormones are leaving us at higher risk of health problems like osteoporosis and cardiovascular disease, our moods are all over the place, and our bodies are primed for putting on weight around the middle.

No brainer: six reasons why you need to get exercising NOW:

Tackles the middle-age spread.[1]

Keeps your bones strong.[2]

Keeps your mind alert.[3]

Protects your heart.[4]

Boosts your mood.[5]

Helps you sleep.[6]

HOW MUCH SHOULD I BE EXERCISING?

The general advice is that you should be exercising for half an hour a day, five days a week.[7] I'd say that as a starting point you should aim to exercise a minimum of three times a week, then see how you get on.[7]

Grab one of those weekly planners and at the start of each week, sit down and plan exercise into your diary. Say to yourself, 'right, this is exercise time' and book in some slots. Then put that planner somewhere you just can't ignore it, like a pinboard or on your fridge.

Look at your week as a whole and plot in the best times for you. You could schedule in exercise every Monday, Wednesday and Friday and give yourself the weekend off, for example. Or if you know Mondays are bad because they are full-on workwise and you just won't commit, go for another day instead.

YOU ARE NEVER TOO BUSY TO EXERCISE

No excuses! You always have time to exercise. Once you start making time for it, you'll be amazed how it soon becomes part of your life. If you find yourself thinking, 'I work so hard that I don't have time during the day', or 'all I want to do at the end of the day is collapse onto the sofa', then I've got the simplest of fixes: just get up earlier.

Set your alarm for half an hour earlier, get your workout out of the way first thing and you'll still have all that time for everything else you need to fit in during the day.

I used to do a class at 7am every Monday morning and I was so smug for having the first workout of the week crossed off the list by 7.45am. I always used to post a really smug selfie of me with a caption like 'oooh, exercise – tick'. I mean, I literally *hated* myself for posting it, but at the same time I felt so good to have it all done and it really set me up for the week ahead.

FIND AN EXERCISE THAT YOU LIKE

People often ask me for my best exercise tips, and absolute top of the list is *find something you like*.

[1] NHS.uk (2019), 'Benefits of exercise', https://www.nhs.uk/live-well/exercise/exercise-health-benefits/

[2] NHS.uk (2019), 'Osteoporosis: prevention', https://www.nhs.uk/conditions/osteoporosis/prevention/

[3] NHS.uk (2019), 'Benefits of exercise', https://www.nhs.uk/live-well/exercise/exercise-health-benefits/

[4] British Heart Foundation, 'Physical Inactivity', https://www.bhf.org.uk/informationsupport/risk-factors/physical-inactivity

[5] NHS.uk (2019), 'Benefits of exercise', https://www.nhs.uk/live-well/exercise/exercise-health-benefits/

[6] B.A. Dolezal et al. (2017), 'Interrelationship between Sleep and Exercise: A Systematic Review', Advances in Preventive Medicine, doi.org/10.1155/2017/1364387

[7] NHS.uk (2021), 'Physical activity guidelines for adults aged 19 to 64', https://www.nhs.uk/live-well/exercise/exercise-guidelines/physical-activity-guidelines-for-adults-aged-19-to-64/

Don't go and do something just because you feel you should. If it makes you feel uncomfortable or you think it's boring, you just won't stick to it. People will say to me 'I'm trying to run every day but I absolutely hate it' and I think, well, why are you doing it? It's the same if you hate spin with a passion. Even though you think you *should* be doing a 6am class because it's good cardio, don't waste your money, because you won't stick to it in the long run.

If you haven't exercised for a while or you want to switch things up, try something new. It could be Zumba or swimming, it could be workouts at home, or you could try spin or running and just love it. The trick is to experiment and try lots of different things.

At the risk of sounding like an advert – but this is my book so I reckon I can definitely promote my fitness platform! – there are over 500 different workouts on my fitness platform, which is called www. ownyourgoalsdavina.com. You can just try loads of different workouts and see what you like. The workouts vary from five minutes to fifty minutes, and there's food on there, and special menopause programmes – there are so many things for you to explore. And there are some really nice wellbeing articles, too.

GETTING STARTED, OR SHORT ON TIME? TRY HOME WORKOUTS

It massively came into its own during Covid, but I think working out at home is fantastic at any time. The option of being able to just hit play in your bedroom or living room and fit in a workout in between other tasks without even needing to leave the house is just so handy.

It's also brilliant if you don't fancy a group class or going to the gym, or the weather is horrible outside. If you are feeling shy, embarrassed about sweating, your age, your size or you just don't feel very sociable, it's a great way to keep up the momentum in a safe space. There are loads of home workouts to choose from: Own Your Goals Davina, there are lots of free videos on YouTube and of course there's the lovely Joe Wicks, too.

WHY WALKING IS EPIC

It's so underrated and overlooked, but I love walking. It's free, it doesn't need loads of fancy equipment and it totally clears my head. It's also so easy to build into your life. Try walking the kids to school, walking to the shops or the train station, instead of jumping into the car.

I'm out walking twice a day with my dog Bo – I wear a running belt over my clothes that my kids laugh at, but it's brilliant because I pop my dog treats and poo bags in there and get walking.

This leads me straight to another tip: if you love animals and have space for them in your life, get a dog. Trust me, you won't regret it. Dogs are just so wonderfully unconditional with their love and make the BEST companions!

A dog really doesn't care if you're feeling menopausal, they just need to get a bloody walk. It's like having your own canine Mr Motivator, minus the spandex – I'm out with Bo twice a day, come rain or shine.

Walking is a brilliant weight-bearing exercise that helps to build bone strength. Basically, a weight-bearing exercise is where you work against gravity, so if walking isn't your bag, dancing or even climbing the stairs also count.

One last thing about walking. Remember the mantra from the start of the book about 'walking with purpose'? Well, kick it up a gear and walk faster. Putting a little spring in your step will mean you get to where you want to go quicker, you'll burn more calories, get your heart rate up and those endorphins going. I'll often put my AirPods in and get my power-walk on with Bo keeping up alongside me. I might look a bit mad and give other walkers a giggle, but who cares? I love it.

So next time you are out for a walk, remember: head up, shoulders back, tummy tight, swing those arms and get walking.

LIVE NEAR WATER? TRY WILD SWIMMING

Wild swimming – that's swimming in lakes, ponds, outdoor pools and the sea – is having something of a moment right now. And with good reason: studies show a cold dip can boost your immune system and metabolism, improve sleep and mood, which is why cold water therapy is so good for you.[8]

A while ago I saw a clip on the news about a group of women who go cold-water swimming together in Swansea, South Wales, to help with their menopause symptoms.

Wearing swimming cozzies, wetsuits and beanies, they ran into the sea and took the plunge, freezing their bits off, shrieking at the cold, but letting out these huge belly laughs. The chat, the camaraderie and the exercise, it looked brilliant.

WHY A KITCHEN DISCO MIGHT BE JUST WHAT YOU NEED

Exercise doesn't always have to be cross-country running in all weathers or lifting weights down the gym. Fitting in twenty minutes here or half an hour of exercise there can and *does* make all the difference.

That can be any activity that gets you moving, too – going for a walk, playing with the kids or grandkids in the park, and then, my personal favourite, dancing to some bangers in the kitchen.

All activity counts; whatever you choose to do, you'll still be lapping everyone

[8] B. Knechtle et al. (2020) 'Cold water swimming-benefits and risks: a narrative review', International Journal of Environmental Research and Public Health, doi.org/10.3390/ijerph17238984

who's lolling on the sofa watching Netflix and eating crisps.

YOU DON'T HAVE TO GO IT ALONE – GET A WORKOUT BUDDY

If willpower is an issue, get yourself an 'excuse buddy'. Whether a friend, partner or workmate at lunchtime, having someone else to be accountable to is a big kick up the backside, motivation-wise. You'll be less likely to cry off if you just don't fancy it and it'll be loads more fun.

I go running with my mate Anna. She's a bit younger than me, and she's a much better runner. She's very motivating and she's extremely kind – if I've got a bit un-running-fit for a while, she will always do a run-walk with me, even though she could run a half marathon at any given moment.

She's also a great motivator for me because she calls me up and goes, 'I'm going to go for a run, do you want to come?' And I'll be thinking, 'Dammit, I thought I'd got away with it...'. But especially in the holidays when I'm around a bit more – in the term-time it's quite difficult – she's fantastic at getting me out and doing something with her. I find her so inspiring.

And look, sometimes she might be going for a run and she inspires me to go for a run at home if I can't go all the way over to her house. I might think,

well she's done a run, I'm going to, too. So you don't have to do it face-to-face if that isn't feasible; you could do an online workout together; you don't even have to be in the same time zone.

Another good thing to do is set up a weekly catch-up to review your goals with your workout buddy and plan ahead for the next week.

CHOOSE A WORKOUT TO SUIT YOUR MOOD

Interpretive dance to the strains of Enya isn't going to cut it if all you want to do is pogo around and listen to Rage Against the Machine very, very loudly.

If I'm in a bad mood then I'll choose a workout to really push those feelings out, like a boxing class. I whack the drum and bass on and really get it out of my system. Try it – I can guarantee you'll feel tons better afterwards.

On the flip side, if you are feeling sad or fragile, then do something that's gentle or loving, like Pilates or some nice yoga stretches.

It is also brilliant to be involved in charity challenges, which will increase your motivation – try the Couch to 5k, or just sign up to a charity walk with a group.

EAT YOUR WAY TO A HEALTHIER MENOPAUSE

I often get asked about weight control in midlife... I'm not a dietitian, but my experience has been that I just do not burn the same number of calories the older I get. So to offset that I still eat the same foods I always have, just a little less of them. I don't obsessively calorie count. Come on, let's be honest, life is too short.

Food can be a big emotional crutch for those points in life when it feels like everything is getting overwhelming. I know I'm not alone in having eaten my feelings during the Covid lockdowns. Menopause can be one of those times, too. You're too knackered to cook something wholesome, you've had a bad day at work, you're generally feeling at a low ebb, and that massive slab of chocolate sitting in the cupboard, practically winking at you, looks way too tempting to pass up on. Just a few squares turns into a whole family-sized bar within minutes.

I have found that my metabolism at this stage of my life has naturally slowed down a bit, and I do find it harder to lose weight if I put on a few pounds. The way I keep on top of things is by being active and being sensible with what I eat. I'm not restrictive in terms of diet, I just make sure that I am sensible for a few days if I know I've been pigging out and eating that little bit more.

If you are in a position where you know the weight has crept up on you for whatever reason, to achieve meaningful weight loss you need a two-pronged attack, twenty per cent exercise and eighty per cent food.

SPARE TYRE? DON'T PANIC

Weight gain in midlife is not inevitable and if you want to, you can lose it.

Our muscle mass reduces during menopause, so we need to keep eating plenty of protein. But if you keep eating at the rate you did when you were in your twenties you can put on weight without realising it.

If you need to cut back, the first place to start is looking at your portion sizes. You don't need a big, fancy set of scales in the kitchen, you can just use your hand as a guide.

Size of your palm - serving of protein like lean meat or fish

Size of your fist - serving of veg

One cupped hand - serving of carbs

One thumb - serving of fats

GET YOURSELF A SMALLER PLATE

Another really easy tip I use after I've been over-indulging – this one comes into its own after Christmas – is switching to a smaller plate.

You might feel hungry for a bit, but once you start to lose weight and your stomach shrinks a little, then you will start to need less food.

BE HONEST ABOUT THOSE OCCASIONAL TREATS

I've seen kids go to university who in their first year will literally put on anything up to a stone in weight and it's purely from the alcohol and the fast food at four o'clock in the morning. In America they even have a nickname for it: the Freshman 15.

I'm not saying you have to ditch all the things you love, just don't go overboard and have your favourite takeaway three times a week, or have a double helping at every meal. Moderation is the key here.

Sugar is my nemesis. Once I start, I find it really hard to stop. Sometimes I'll buy chocolate and other treats 'for Chester' knowing FULL WELL that really they are for me.

If you do something similar and end up polishing off all the treats all the time, then it might be better to just clear them out from the cupboards until

you can forge some better habits. Out of sight, out of mind.

Obviously I don't drink any more, but if you've found yourself getting into the habit of a couple of glasses of wine every night, then make a pact with yourself to either drop the weeknight vino altogether or limit it to fewer nights a week. Alcohol is full of empty calories and it's a real barrier to getting a good night's sleep.

WILL HRT MAKE ME <u>LOSE</u> WEIGHT?

There's nothing in HRT that makes you lose weight per se, but you will probably find that if you have a few pounds to lose, HRT will give you the impetus to do something about it. I mean, fatigue, anxiety, depression and aches and pains are enough to drain the motivation from the most committed gym-goer. For me, I've found that HRT has helped with my symptoms and so helps with reigniting my desire to get active.

THE KEY VITAMINS AND NUTRIENTS YOU NEED TO SEE YOU THROUGH MENOPAUSE AND BEYOND

Calcium

Calcium keeps bones strong and healthy and is believed to protect against osteoporosis. You should be able to get the calcium you need from green leafy veg, tofu, bony fish like salmon, dairy products and plant-based milks and cereals that have been fortified with calcium.[9]

Vitamin D

This vitamin helps our bodies absorb calcium, but it's hard to get all we need from just our food. Most of our vitamin D will come from exposure to sunlight during sunnier months, but you might also want to think about taking a vitamin D supplement as a good insurance policy – especially in the autumn and winter months. Taking 1,000iu daily has been shown to improve bone health, insulin sensitivity and immunity.[10]

Magnesium

Magnesium is a mineral that can improve sleep, lower stress and soothe sore muscles. You should be able to get all the magnesium you need from your diet – nuts like almonds and cashews are a brilliant source, as well as green veg and wholegrains – but bear in mind that things like alcohol and caffeine can affect absorption.[11]

Others

The supplements that I take daily are a combined vitamin C and vitamin D tablet. I have a chewy one, which I really like because it tastes like a sweet! I also take a multivitamin B (so all the vitamin Bs in one), and in the evening I take a magnesium to help me sleep and to look after all my muscles. And I also take collagen daily. Collagen is full of protein, so it's improving my protein intake, too, which is great. I actually take collagen not just for hair, skin and nails (which is what lots of people take it for) but for my insides – my tendons and ligaments.

You should always talk to your doctor.

---

[9] NHS.uk (2021), 'Vitamins and minerals: calcium', https://www.nhs.uk/conditions/vitamins-and-minerals/calcium/

[10] NHS.uk (2021), 'Vitamins and minerals: vitamin D', https://www.nhs.uk/conditions/vitamins-and-minerals/vitamin-d/

[11] NHS.uk (2021): Vitamins and minerals: others', https://www.nhs.uk/conditions/vitamins-and-minerals/others/

SKINCARE SOS

Parched, wrinkled and a bit sad.

Sounds like I'm describing a lonesome raisin, but that was actually what my skin looked like during perimenopause.

I love seeing people's eyes crinkle when they smile, but the wrinkles that were staring back at me in the mirror in the mornings got me down.

If you've experienced the same, help is at hand: enter the undisputed queen of skincare, Caroline Hirons.

Caroline is a globally qualified advanced aesthetician, trained in well over a hundred brands. Her career involves bespoke facials and training teams internationally for top brands. She has decades of experience in the skincare industry and is an absolute force of nature. I first started following Caroline on social media and it was like finding a skincare spirit animal. She's honest, upfront and when it comes to menopausal skincare, she gets it. She rails against the whole industry that has sprung up around menopause – or moneypause, as she calls it – and what she doesn't know about skincare just isn't worth knowing. She's a bona fide menopause warrior, and she's here to talk us through what you need to know about peri- and menopausal skincare.

Then, once she's shared her wisdom, I've got some tips on a completely no-fuss make-up routine that literally takes five minutes to do and I promise will make you feel great.

So, right now I'm going to hand over to Caroline Hirons to tell you why your skin is changing, and for her expert tips on what you can do to make it look and feel great.

CAROLINE HIRON'S
SKINCARE MASTERCLASS

WHAT'S GOING ON WITH MY SKIN DURING PERIMENOPAUSE?

When the oestrogen levels start to fluctuate during perimenopause, it can have a knock-on effect on your skin. The falling oestrogen will affect your skin's ability to retain ceramides, fatty acids that help the skin lock in moisture.

Everyone's skin reacts differently – you might have no issues at all, but for many women, perimenopause means being prone to redness and spotty skin. When I turned forty, I developed adult acne out of nowhere. I had what I would call the 'heavy-duty' spots that never come to a head and linger like a volcano that just wouldn't erupt, especially around the chin area.

Because your skin is literally becoming thinner, you'll also probably notice (and this is the case from perimenopause onwards) that it takes longer for the skin to heal, so if you do get a spot, it'll take longer to go away. Your skin will be slower to respond because it doesn't have the same receptors to deal with spots, and this goes for cuts or open wounds, which will probably take longer to heal as well.

What to do about it

Don't jump on the latest trendy ingredient or start buying a whole load of products aimed at ageing skin. 'Ageing skin' is about taking care of wrinkles, but in perimenopause usually the main things you need to address are redness and spots.

Having said that, you don't want to aggressively treat your whole face by throwing the kitchen sink at it. Please, don't attack your face! Sometimes when women get spots they start treating their skin like it's the enemy. Treat the areas where the spots are, but not your whole face.

When I was perimenopausal I switched from a heavier moisturiser to a lighter, water-based one that penetrates the skin quickly. It felt a lot lighter and more comfortable on the skin.

Look for products with ceramides and peptides. Peptides are amino acids that can help boost dull and dehydrated skin. Both ceramides and peptides are a gentle way to keep your skin barrier in check without being super-aggressive.

MENOPAUSE AND SKIN

As you move into menopause, oestrogen depletes further and your skin starts to lose its tone and elasticity, leading to wrinkles and jowls. If you find your skin has switched from being spotty to feeling tight and dry after cleansing, it might be a sign of oestrogen falling further and that you are heading closer to menopause.

And, to add fuel to the fire, it becomes harder for your skin to retain moisture, so you might find your skin switches from spotty to dry, flaky and itchy and you are left thinking, what the hell is this?

Because hormones are still fluctuating as you enter menopause, you can get the odd zinger of a spot, but in general your skin tends to be drier and more sallow-looking at this stage.

What to do about it

Unless it's come on prescription from a medical professional, save your money and give a wide berth to products that promise to stop hot flushes or that will 'fix' your menopausal skin.

If your skin is dry and dull-looking, the key thing is getting moisture back in. That doesn't mean you have to go for a really rich moisturiser (unless your skin is feeling very dry and itchy), as something water-based can work just as well.

Don't go and spend a fortune on a clay detox mask, do the opposite – look for a hydrating mask. And if you've got a big event coming up, a good facial oil can fix a thousand sins very quickly.

Again, look for products with ceramides and peptides. Think gentle and reassuring products that aren't going to throw your skin into a hissy fit. For daytime, menopausal skin will often respond well to cleansing milks and creams, facial mists and a good moisturiser – and don't skip a good SPF to protect your skin! The general rule of thumb is that if you can read a book outside in natural light, then you need to use SPF. At night, repeat your daytime routine, without applying the SPF.

I also find that I'm not good with active products anymore, like retinols. My skincare barrier is permanently depleted because of menopause, so it doesn't like a really strong retinol that I would have been able to tolerate five or ten years ago. The main thing is to listen to your skin and what it can cope with.

NO-FUSS, FIVE-MINUTE MAKE-UP ROUTINE

When I was in my forties, I started putting on a little bit of make-up every day. Even if it's just doing my lashes in a rush before setting out, it makes me happy and feel good.

My make-up artist, Cheryl Phelps-Gardiner, who I first met on a Garnier shoot, is AMAZING. She's worked with all the great photographers, like David Bailey, and has worked with all the supermodels, too. Cheryl was the first person to tell me that unless you are going for a full-on dramatic smoky eye, don't put eyeliner or anything on the lower lids: it is very ageing as it pulls your eyes down.

Here are some of her top bits of advice.

ESSENTIAL MAKE-UP TIPS FROM CHERYL PHELPS-GARDINER

This is for all women who want their make-up to be super-fast and super-easy. As we get older, our skin loses the bloom of youth, and that's where I can help you recreate that. So there's no Kim Kardashian tips to be found here. I have made recommendations for specific brands, but there are plenty of other options available out there.

FOUNDATION

There are many choices of foundation: liquid, cream, powder-based, water-based.

What I find the best and easiest to use is Chanel Vitalumiere liquid foundation, which has a light to medium coverage. It has a nice light-reflecting sheen and also comes in a good range of colours. It is a bit pricey, but you really only need a small amount, so it will last a long time.

If you have good skin you can skip foundation – for instance, Davina has great skin, and if she is doing her own make-up for work she will often use tinted moisturiser instead (Laura

Mercier have some great shades).

No matter what type of skin you have, less is more. Ignore dark spots or blemishes at this stage, to keep the skin looking fresh. You are aiming for a thin veil over the face and down the neck.

CONCEALER

It's a good idea to choose a palette that has two or more shades so you can mix the exact colour of the skin surrounding the blemish. Bobbi Brown, Laura Mercier and Il Makiage do them – in fact, most make-up brands have palettes. I like the yellow tones over the pink tones, and using a brush like a lipstick brush gives you more control to mix and apply rather than using your fingertips.

Under the eyes I use YSL Touche Éclat and Secret Brightening powder by Laura Mercier... this is a MUST in my kit, it's a very fine light-reflecting powder, and I think it's magic! Laura Mercier also do a brush called the Pony Tail, which is perfect for applying a delicate, light touch of powder to blemishes and under the eyes.

CHEEKS

So once you have the flawless foundation, now we need to put back that bloom.

You want to emulate the colour of your cheeks if you had just enjoyed a brisk walk on a fresh winter morning, which is pink with plum undertones.

I go straight to Boomstick Colour, as it's the perfect shade. It looks terrifyingly dark burgundy in the packaging, but it's not, it gives a veil of colour akin to blushing and magically fits every skin tone. It's also great on lips, with a wonderful

sheen. But whatever blusher you use, make it a cream one.

Then you need to add an extra bit of sheen to the top of the cheek bones, the tip of the nose and a little to the centre of the chin. I like Total Euphoria by NARS, but again there are many brands that do gloss sticks. You want a glow, but no sparkle – you are looking for fresh, dewy skin with a flush of colour... Oh, and don't forget lashings of mascara.

HAIR TO THE RESCUE

Good hair, for me, is a real confidence boost. Like putting on a bit of lippy, if my hair looks good then I *feel* good and just on it.

I first started going grey when I was twenty-five and I've been dyeing it ever since (actually, I have been colouring my own hair since I was eighteen, but this was just in order to get rid of my pesky greys). I know loads of women look incredibly chic with grey hair but I'm just not quite ready to embrace the greys.

I will occasionally have my hair coloured on a shoot, but it does surprise people that I really do colour my hair myself at home. It's just more convenient for me than sitting at the hairdresser for three hours. I can whack it on, chat to the kids or get a bit of work done while waiting for the colour to work its magic.

When I hit perimenopause and pre-HRT, my hair felt a bit flat, dry and meh. I know now that my hair was crying out for hormones.

Michael Douglas is a session hairdresser who has been in the business for over thirty years. What he doesn't know about hair isn't worth knowing. He's worked with all the huge brands, he's worked in advertising, commercials, films, TV shows. He's done many celebrities' hair and has been my hairdresser for over twenty years. He does these hair clinics on his Instagram page, which are Instagram lives, where he invites women and men to come on and he solves their hair problems – including many menopausal women.

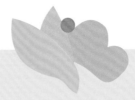

MICHAEL'S HAIR MASTERCLASS

Here are some of the fantastic tips that he gives to menopausal women on his Instagram lives.

FOUR REASONS YOUR HAIR SUFFERS DURING PERIMENOPAUSE AND MENOPAUSE

The natural ageing process

As we get older, our cell production slows down and our cells are reproduced from their previous version. I read a brilliant analogy in a scientific paper that explains this: it's a bit like when you make a photocopy. The first time you photocopy an image it's crisp and clear, but when you photocopy a photocopy again and again it's not the same. And that's essentially how our cells age.

In addition, the quality and amount of hair you have deteriorates as the follicle (which anchors each hair into the skin) starts to get older. It stops producing colour, so you can get more greys and the hair itself becomes thinner.

Hormones

Hormones play an enormous role in the health of our hair throughout our lives.

To break it down into really simple terms, our hair goes through a growing phase and a shedding phase. Our hair is in the growing phase about ninety per cent of the time and the rest in the shedding phase – this is when you might run your fingers through your hair and a few strands come loose, or you maybe notice hair collecting in the bottom of the shower.

But the fall in oestrogen during perimenopause and menopause can throw this all off balance. That drop in oestrogen slows down that growing phase from ninety per cent to sixty per cent and ramps up the shedding phase so you get more hair loss and less hair growth.

With oestrogen in retreat, it means androgens that are usually suppressed become more prominent, and one of the first things they will do is shrink the hair follicles. Your hair will grow, but it will be much finer.

Your genes

Female pattern baldness, where the crown area is usually affected, is a hereditary condition in which the growing phase is shorter. It can happen at any age, but is most common after menopause, when the hormone changes also affect the length of the growing phase.

Diet

The slowing down of the growing phase is largely related to hormones, but it's also connected to health and diet. Your hair is pretty low down the priority list when it comes to getting all the vitamins and nutrients from your diet. Your muscles, bones, teeth, eyes and skin get first dibs, so if you aren't eating a balanced diet, then your hair won't get what it needs.

TIPS ON HOW TO TACKLE HAIR PROBLEMS DURING MENOPAUSE

If you're in menopause, going through a shedding phase and your diet isn't great then, blimey, your hair is going to be suffering – and it will show.

Here are some options on how to get your hair back to its best.

See a doctor about your hormones

Putting the oestrogen back will help to re-establish the growing and shedding phase. You need to stick with it, though, as you won't see a massive improvement in your hair overnight. Hair grows on average a centimetre each month, so you need to be patient and give it at least 4–6 months before you see the real effects of HRT.

Don't ever underestimate the power of a healthy diet

We are so bloody busy fitting everything in that we often forget to re-fuel and eat properly. Our hair type is in the genes, so you can't make fine hair grow back thicker, or curly hair grow straight, but protein is a wonderful way to make your hair grow back better. You need about 55–60g of protein in your diet a day to help grow healthy new hair. Collagen supplements containing amino acids (a type of protein) are great for hair, nails and skin. Vitamin D also helps to keep the hair in the growing phase, so make sure you are getting your daily amount. Iron also helps to keep the hair in the growing phrase.

Give your hair some quick oomph

A couple of clip-in hair extensions can really help create the appearance of thicker, fuller hair.

Root touch-up sprays are good to put on any patchy areas as a tiny bit of powdered colour.

Look after your scalp

The scalp is super-important – it's the fertile seed bed to grow a good head of hair.

If you are suffering from hair loss you could try using a scalp dermabrasion treatment, which cleans the scalp and helps to prepare the follicles to grow hair. Be sure to go to a specialist for this.

If you have female pattern hair loss, then at-home treatments with the ingredient minoxidil can help to re-awaken the hair follicles that have already died. You massage it into the scalp every day and it can yield some great results. Again, it won't make thin hair thicker, because that's down to your genes.

Give your hair some TLC

If you blow-dry, curl or straighten your hair regularly, then you need to be using products such as hair protection cream or blow-dry spray on wet hair before you get to work.

Less is more when it comes to straightening; people use irons way too much, dragging them through the same section three or four times. It's better to do it once, slowly, with some product on to protect the hair.

While you're at it, have a look at the brushes you are using. Brushes have a shelf life, so if they are looking a bit tired and broken, replace them.

Don't let your age define your 'do'

I really don't buy into the idea that your hair needs to look a certain way once you reach a certain age. You are never too old for the style you want. What you want is the best possible version of you.

One of my clients is the EastEnders' actress Ann Mitchell. She's in her eighties and looks fantastic.

FIVE WAYS TO MAKE YOU LOOK AND FEEL YOUNGER

SMILE!

It's that simple!

Smiling makes you seem warm, positive, approachable, and just someone people will want to be around. Smiling is also super-sexy, too.

When you are smiling, even though it gives you loads of wrinkles around your eyes, people are so busy looking at your big gorgeous grin they won't notice a couple of crow's feet.

GET YOUR TEETH DONE

Balding men will often ask Michael for advice when they don't know what to do about losing their hair and he always says to them: 'get your teeth done.'

And it is so, so true. You really can't underestimate the power of a lovely set of gnashers. People LOVE seeing a lovely big smile, and getting your teeth fixed is a huge confidence boost.

It was seeing my kids get braces that inspired me to do it. It totally transformed the way they smiled and carried themselves.

So I thought I'd have a bit of that too, and I got Invisalign® braces. They're completely clear and help to straighten your teeth, and they've made such a difference. Also, it's worth saying I was in my fifties when I had them fitted – so there's no age limit.

HITCH UP THOSE PUPPIES!

When we get older, especially if we've had babies, our boobs start going south. They are suddenly not in the place they were before. And we all start letting those bra straps get longer and loooonger, sometimes to the point where it looks like we're wearing braces, not a sodding bra.

Don't do it. Tighten those bra straps and lift up those puppies. Your boobs will still look great, they just need some extra support and oomph.

And while you're at it, go through your knicker and bra drawer and chuck out those bras that have seen better days. I remember reading a survey that said women stuck to wearing the same two bras for a decade. TEN years! Think of all the action and hormone changes your breasts have gone through over the space of a decade – not to mention how many washing-machine cycles your bras have been put through.

If your once-white bras are greying, you know what to do: Chuck. Them. Out.

Go and get fitted, buy something new – whether it's comfy, sexy, supportive, whatever – and bring a bit of cleavage back into your life.

NO MORE GROANING

Have you found yourself starting to make 'oooof', 'eeeee' and 'urghhhhhh' sounds when you bend down to pick something up? It's like the clarion call of old age.

Over the last few years, whenever I would bend down to take off my trainers I would hear myself make similar groaning sounds and it instantly made me feel like I was five hundred years old. I mean, I don't remember making those sorts of sounds in my thirties, and I've had to train myself to bite my lip and not do it.

If you've been doing it too, Stop. DON'T GROAN!

WALK WITH PURPOSE

Young people walk like they are going somewhere, and I noticed as I got older that my walking just slowed down so much. I thought, *God, I've stopped looking like I'm going somewhere*. But not only that, you kind of slow down and you're not burning as many calories as you would have done when you were younger.

So just remember to keep that pace up, because doing that is exercise, and it makes you look younger – or appear younger – and it gives you those endorphins, which we love. Put on some tunes in your ears and crack out the bangers! That will get you picking up the pace.

ONE LAST THING: DON'T FORGET TO LOVE YOURSELF

As a group, we menopausal women are so hard on ourselves. I mean, I guess women are often hard on themselves their entire lives, but we spend so much time being critical of ourselves – and, indeed, of others. When I get judgmental of other women, I always think, 'Ok, what's going on with *me*?' Because if I'm judgmental of other women, then there is usually, sure as hell, something going on with me that I either need to talk about with some friends, or get off my chest.

We've all got enough to get on with in the world. Think about all the things that women, throughout history and in our own lives, have to endure: birth, periods, hairy legs, menopause … all of those things. We DON'T NEED to bitch about each other and judge other women. Let's not do it!

We need to remember, menopausal ladies, that we are in our second spring, and this is an opportunity to cast off our previous personas, and looks, and ideals, and figure out this new phase in our lives – a phase that can last for thirty, forty years – where we can totally reinvent ourselves and become who we want to be.

If you eat your bodyweight in cake one day and you haven't exercised for a while, or you're just annoyed with yourself because you haven't achieved what you hoped to achieve, it's ok. Just press the reset button and say to yourself, *ok, tomorrow's another day and we can start after that.*

Embrace your body. Don't get me wrong, I often wish I had legs like Elle Macpherson, or boobs that hadn't fed three babies, but I do love my body. We've been through a lot together. It's been pregnant three times, it's been battered, it's been through sporting madness, it's yo-yo'd a lot, weight-wise. But it's mine.

Let's celebrate our body shapes. I know that the menopause chucks a lot at us, physically and mentally, but you know what? We're all still here and we're still standing … just! Hahahaha.

Believe me when I say to you: I see you. And you look fucking great.

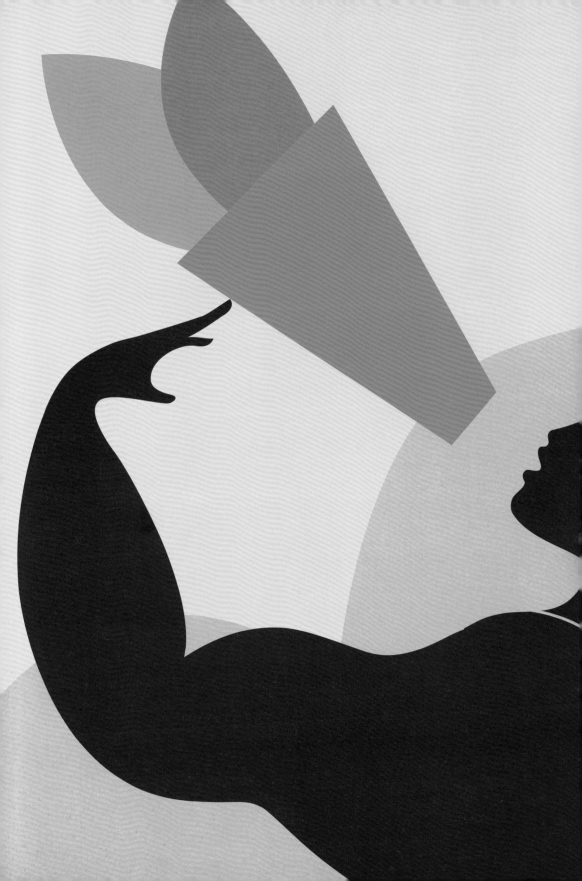

CHAPTER 14

LET'S RECLAIM THE CHANGE AND SPREAD THE MENOPAUSING MESSAGE

I hate the word menopause.

It means 'final period'. It sounds like a full stop. Menopause and then ... nothing. A black hole of boredom. An abyss.

But in Japan they call the menopause the second spring. I bloody love that! Not the autumn, not the fucking winter, the *second spring,* people.

I might sound like a bit of an old hippy, but once you get your hormones in check, there comes a rebirth. Once we start getting levelled out, that is the time when we can really start living again.

Rather than signalling the end of life, our menopause is our midlife, our mid-point. If you were born back in 1841, you would have only expected to live until the age of forty-two. These days, the average life expectancy for women in England is eighty-three.[1]

See?!! We have SO MUCH more living to do.

When you kiss goodbye to your baby-making years there is a sort of liberation where you think to yourself, what do *I* want? What's next for *me*?

For me, I'm in a good place now. My hormones are relatively ok. Career-wise, I'm in a happy place. I'm in a happy place with all of my relationships – my friends, my family, my partner. And now my kids are getting older, I just love watching them mature and grow – not just physically, obviously, but mentally, too – and turn into young adults.

And I'll tell you another thing I absolutely love; I love seeing other women embracing this midlife freedom – making changes, trying new things, maybe starting businesses, ridding themselves of inhibitions and outdated labels and getting out there in the world.

Society ignores menopausal and post-menopausal women at its peril. We are feisty, funny, sexy, wise, and we aren't going anywhere.

We've got to reclaim 'the change' and turn the phrase on its head. Menopause isn't about ageing and slowing down, but about moving on to the next phase of our lives, where we can strike out and do the things we want for *us*.

WHY WE ALL NEED TO BE MORE GOLDIE

I can literally lose hours scrolling through social media, and one of my favourites is Goldie Hawn's Instagram account.

Goldie makes me absolutely howl. There's a brilliant clip of her jumping around like a maniac while doing a trampoline workout – if you haven't seen it, go watch it now. I was out of breath just watching her.

[1] The Kings Fund (2021), 'What is happening to life expectancy in England?' https://www.kingsfund.org.uk/publications/whats-happening-life-expectancy-england

What I love about her is her incredible
energy. She's in her seventies, looks
amazing, does what she wants, says
what she wants and doesn't give a stuff
what people think.

We all need to be more Goldie. We need
to be inspired by women who are ten,
twenty, thirty years ahead of us, who
can tell us it's going to be ok, and that
midlife isn't about being buttoned up
and acting our age, but about shedding
our inhibitions. And don't forget, ladies,
that YOU are ten, twenty, thirty years
ahead of other young women, and it's
up to YOU to be the inspiration for
them. To show them that it's all going
to be ok.

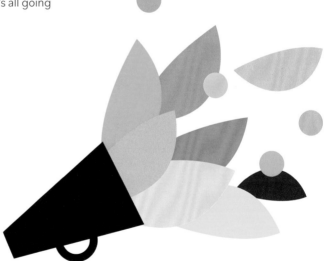

MENOPAUSING WOMEN WHO ARE ABSOLUTELY KILLING IT

When you scroll through social media, you quickly get the message that there are so many women out there who are going through the same thing as you, and so many women have reached out to tell their stories to me, too. These women are all brilliant and helping to get the conversation started.

'I'm sharing my menopause journey to show others not to be embarrassed or ashamed.' — Linzi

Linzi is forty-seven, perimenopausal and had to navigate the loss of a sibling to suicide during lockdown, as well as raising four-year-old twins and managing a chronic illness.

Menopause could be a huge inconvenience BUT I'm actually learning to move with it rather than against it. Davina's wellbeing posts have inspired me to take more care of my body as I was only focusing on my mind/brain health previously.

I know the importance of educating myself, talking and sharing the menopause journey with others and not to be embarrassed about it or ashamed.

Many of my friends are still in their thirties, so I want to be an example for them to see that it's nothing to be scared of.

I've never been one to do much exercise but now I'm setting up a running club in my local community in Tunbridge Wells, starting daily rides on my Peloton bike and increasing my exposure to the outdoors every day for maximum vitamin D. I have also changed my diet to focus more on 'living' foods and less alcohol. The results are already making a huge difference. I could just feel sorry for myself or I could get up and take ownership for my life as a woman – and I'm most certainly doing the latter. I feel blessed to be able to go through this and become stronger as a result.

Hey, Linzi – what? You're setting up a running club in Tunbridge Wells? WHERE? I wanna come!

'I felt like me again.' — Adele

Adele is the owner and CEO of two businesses that employ more than forty staff and have a combined £3 million turnover. As she says in her own words, she's one busy woman.

Since the age of forty-two things were not 'right' – super-heavy periods, memory problems and bowel issues before my period. My moods changed daily.

Seeing my GP, I was told I had IBS or depression. Not once was the menopause discussed. My 1970s Catholic-school education meant female biology was covered very quickly in lessons, and I didn't join the dots as I still thought of myself as being too young to be menopausal.

By the time I was forty-six, I was having the same symptoms as above but also started to have itchy skin. I often had a swollen stomach, and my memory and speech ability were so bad that my health suffered and my anxiety went through the roof.

I started to self-diagnose with Dr Google and actually planned my own funeral, convinced I had cancer. My GP kept testing my bloods, sent me for scans on

the bowel and brain but never tested my hormone levels. I had to cope with these symptoms while running two businesses and handling day-to-day life with a growing and demanding teenage family.

When I asked my GP about menopause, he simply asked if my periods were still happening, and as they were, it was not the menopause, in his opinion. In 2019 a friend suggested seeing a gynaecologist. I was given the details of her doctor and then – BOOM – once scans were completed to rule anything else out, yes, I was perimenopausal. Immediately I was given HRT patches and a progestogen tablet. Within three months, I felt like me again. My ability to communicate in a clear, cohesive manner was back, my ability to stand and talk in public and with confidence came back to allow me to do that.

Adele, showing us that Dr Google is not a good idea! I'm frustrated for you that menopause wasn't flagged up earlier, but I am so glad that you are back to being boss!

'I'm determined we will be the generation to #MakeMenopauseMatter.' — Diane

Diane Danzebrink is a personal therapist and wellbeing consultant specialising in menopause. She is the founder of Menopause Support (menopausesupport.co.uk) and the #MakeMenopauseMatter campaign.

Diane is incredible, an inspiration, and I wanted you to read her story in full, in her own words.

A few years ago, I hadn't given menopause a second thought. Fast-forward to today and I pretty much eat, drink and sleep all things menopause.

In July 2012 I had to have a total hysterectomy, including the removal of both of my ovaries, my womb, and my cervix, as it was suspected that I had ovarian cancer. When somebody tells you that they think you have ovarian cancer you want the surgery done there and then, and waiting for my hospital admission were the longest days of my life.

Following surgery, the gynaecologist explained that the operation had been longer and more complex than expected as she had discovered both severe endometriosis and adenomyosis. That

explained all the heavy, painful periods, pelvic and lower back pain that I had been experiencing for so many years. Unfortunately, my bladder had been damaged during the operation, hence the attractive bag of wee attached to my leg, thankfully only temporary. The good news was that she was quietly confident that my surgery had been done, in her words, 'just in time'; lab results a few weeks later confirmed she was correct, phew!

Prior to my surgery I received no counselling about the potential impacts of being plunged into surgical menopause or the potential symptoms and how to manage them. When I left the hospital, I was simply told to book an appointment with my GP when I felt up to it. I was shocked to hear that there would be no follow up with the gynaecologist.

Many years earlier my mum had been given HRT following her surgery for ovarian cancer, and when I found out that it was derived from pregnant mares' urine I was horrified and decided there and then that HRT would not be for me. The scary stories about HRT and breast cancer did nothing to change my mind. I had no idea just how important replacing hormones was after surgical menopause, as nobody had explained it to me, but I was about to find out.

A few months after surgery things went very wrong, very quickly; physically I was doing well but mentally I was starting to struggle. I was becoming increasingly anxious and losing my confidence. I started to experience panic attacks and I was spending most nights lying awake, desperate for sleep. Sometimes the fear and anxiety would become so overwhelming that I would have to wake my husband to reassure me – not what he needed as he had taken on responsibility for everything as my mental health deteriorated.

Work became completely impossible as I lost confidence, focus and concentration. I was leaving the house less and less and was reluctant to see friends, answer the phone or open post, which I was convinced would only contain bad news. Every day felt darker than the last and getting through them felt like wading through chest-deep treacle. I was becoming increasingly insecure and irrational but continually refused to see the doctor as I thought I was going mad. I was convinced the only way forward was a lifetime of antidepressants or admission to a mental health unit. Finally, my husband had no choice but to ask my mum to come and stay while he went to work, as he had become so concerned about my mental health.

My poor mum looked after me during the day and then was regularly woken during the night when I would creep along the landing, crawl into bed with her and just sob my heart out like a child in an effort not to disturb my poor exhausted husband. The future looked bleak. I felt useless, hopeless and worthless, I had no idea where the real me had disappeared to, I had lost my joy. I felt sad, frightened and lost; I was unrecognisable. What made it all worse is that I have always been the person that others come to for support and advice. The strong, sensible, level-headed friend who can always be relied upon to be a common-sense voice of reason, who could help find a solution to any problem. Where the hell had she disappeared to?

One morning soon after I came very close to taking my own life. I remember thinking what a burden I had become to the people I loved and how it would be better if I was no longer here. I clearly remember the lorry that I was going to put my car into the path of and I would not be here if Henry, one of my Jack Russells, hadn't barked at the right moment and brought me back to reality. I began to sob and shake violently at the thought of what I had almost done. I don't know how I drove home, and I don't remember much about the rest of the day other than telling my husband what I had almost done.

My husband immediately contacted our GP practice and a few hours later I sat in front of the doctor sobbing through the details of the past few months. The doctor explained that I was experiencing severe menopause symptoms due to the drastic reduction of oestrogen caused by the removal of my ovaries. She went on to tell me about the benefits and risks of body identical HRT and how it was different from the HRT my mum had been prescribed. She assured me it was what I needed. The little square patch that she prescribed for me to stick on my thigh twice a week made a difference within a few days and the world no longer felt like such a dark, scary place, but it wasn't long before relief turned to anger.

Looking back at what I had almost done made me wonder how many other women had felt that way due to a lack of the right information and support before menopause came along and threatened to destroy their lives. I remember telling my husband how ludicrous it was that half the population would go through it but none of us ever learn anything about it, and I promised that if I ever felt like me again, I would make damn sure I did something to change the menopause landscape for the future.

It took me about two years to feel like me again. I ended up having to fund a private menopause consultation with a specialist to get the right combination, type and dose of HRT for me. That consultation had to be put on a credit card, and whilst I don't regret it for a moment it angers me that so many women are still being forced to fund private menopause care rather than receiving the help and support they deserve via the NHS. There are millions who could never consider private menopause care, and nor should they

have to, but too many end up suffering in silence and that is a disgrace.

Once I felt stronger, I began to wonder what I could practically do to change things for the future. Many years earlier I had studied counselling but had taken a different career path. I made the decision to go back to studying counselling and coaching and attended professional nurse training in menopause. While I was studying, I set up Menopause Support, which is now a community interest company offering education, information, advice, support and lots of free resources.

Studies completed, I decided to specialise in counselling women experiencing menopause in the hope of helping some of those so desperate for help. I also began to receive requests from the media to speak about the barriers that women faced in accessing the right help and support and the wider effects of menopause on mental health, relationships and careers. My inbox was and always is jammed afterwards with emails from women sharing heartbreaking experiences of how their undiagnosed and untreated menopause symptoms have affected their lives. I am always humbled that complete strangers will share intimate details of their lives in an attempt to get the help they so desperately need.

Life had taken a very unexpected turn, but I was delighted to be able to help raise wider menopause awareness. Coming out of the BBC one morning in

2017, my phone rang and when I answered it the voice at the other end was that of Carolyn Harris MP inviting me to Westminster to offer her help in raising awareness in Parliament. Despite supporting women individually, speaking publicly and working with MPs, it still felt as though I was only scratching the surface, so I decided it was time for a national campaign. In October 2018, with Carolyn's help, I launched the national #MakeMenopauseMatter campaign in Westminster.

The campaign aims are:

→ *To ensure mandatory menopause training for all doctors and medical students.*

→ *To have menopause guidance and support in every workplace.*

→ *To have menopause included in the new RSE curriculum in schools.*

I am delighted to say that thousands have now signed the petition, and just nine months after launching we achieved the aim of having menopause included in the school curriculum in England, with the help of Rachel Maclean MP, which was amazing. However, there is still so much more work to do.

Menopause is not a women's issue; it is a human rights issue. Whilst the majority of those directly affected are women, it can also directly affect transgender and non-binary people, too. It can indirectly affect anybody who knows or loves the

person going through it – partners, families, friends and colleagues.

There is a gaping chasm where menopause education and information should exist. It is just common sense to make menopause education and awareness a priority for our healthcare professionals, business leaders and the public to avoid the breakdown of relationships and families, costs to our health service and to industry, but most importantly to a person's short- and long-term health and wellbeing.

When I decided to start raising awareness publicly back in 2015 it was a very lonely place, as few people were prepared to even say the word menopause. I am delighted that things have changed over the past few years, with many others raising their voices for change. We are certainly moving in the right direction, and I am determined that we will be the generation to #MakeMenopauseMatter.

Thanks so much, Diane. I really wanted to include your story. Keep up the good work! High five!

SPREADING THE
MENOPAUSING MESSAGE

The morning of 28 October 2021 was one of those grey, damp, drizzly days where it felt like the rain would never end.

Wrapped up in a big warm coat, I got off the train at Charing Cross station and walked alone through the wet streets of London. But as I turned into Parliament Square, the setting of countless demos, protests and rallies over the years, the sun broke through the clouds and the biggest grin spread across my face.

YES! I thought. Why? Because on that patch of grass opposite the Houses of Parliament was an army of women who had gathered to take the fight for better menopause care right to the very heart of government.

We were there to support a campaign by Labour MP Carolyn Harris to scrap prescription charges for HRT in England. Placard-waving, t-shirt-wearing, making an absolute bloody racket and refusing to be silent. So many brave, bright, inspiring, BRILLIANT women, all with their own stories to tell.

In the end, the government would not go as far as we wanted, but what it did promise was that women would only pay for their HRT prescription once a year.

It was an amazing result by Carolyn. Standing alongside her and other menopause warriors like Diane Danzebrink, Mariella Frostrup, Penny Lancaster, Sam Evans and Karen Arthur was an incredible feeling.

I cried. I wasn't really even sure why I was crying, but it was an unbelievably emotional time, seeing all these women come together to support a woman, Carolyn Harris, who had a seat in a House that could make things genuinely, really change for women. Not just for us, but for future generations. It was incredibly moving, but I guess what was most significant about that day was that it wasn't about politics or point scoring; it was about women, and effecting change, and the fact that women, men, politicians, campaigners and people from all walks of life were united for one purpose.

'The great thing about this is that it isn't a political matter, this is a women's matter and today everybody came together to make this happen,' I shouted through a megaphone. 'It's not just menopausal women, it's for our daughters … for our grannies who didn't have any support at all.'

On a personal level, it was a real pinch-me moment. It felt like things were really changing for the better. The struggles during my early days of menopause, deciding to speak out and using my platform so others wouldn't feel alone, the incredible response to my documentary, the long nights spent on social media answering questions, offering advice and virtual hugs to women who felt as lost as I once did – that day outside the Houses of Parliament brought it home to me that things ARE changing.

I know that I'm not the first person to bang the drum about menopause. There are so many menopausing warriors out there with fire in their bellies. Peri- and menopausal women need rebranding, to be seen as the funny, sassy, experienced, liberated, boss bitches we are. I never saw myself becoming this woman. The woman with the megaphone. Outside the Houses of bloody Parliament.

But if I can do it, so can you. And we need YOU because we've only just started. You don't need to stand outside the seat of government waving a placard to be a menopausing warrior – although I can recommend it, as it was bloody good fun. We can all play a part in effecting change, in our own way.

We need to get spreading the menopausing message at home, at work, among your mates, or while out walking the dog – and here's how.

No more shame, no more stigma, remember?

BE HONEST

Honest, open conversations are at the heart of this: talking to friends, talking to family, to colleagues, but also with yourself.

My one hope after reading this book is that we can finally consign 'soldiering on', 'putting on a brave face', 'get on with it' type troupes to the bin where they belong. You *know* that you don't have to struggle or put up with things. You know from the stories in this book, or even from personal experience, just how damaging that can be. If you are struggling, speak up and seek help. See a doctor, speak to your friends. Because there IS help out there.

BE AN AMBASSADOR

Use the knowledge you've gained from the pages of this book and talk, talk, talk, TALK about it.

Share this book with your friends, your family, your work colleagues. You don't have to be menopausal. You don't have to be a woman.

Use the information to lobby your workplace for proper support. And if you *are* the boss, then what are you waiting for?

BE AN ALLY

What's that mantra from the military? No man left behind. Well, we want *no one* to be left behind.

It might be an unspoken hunch that something is wrong during a meet up with a mate. Or you spot someone on social media who is having a tough time. Reach out and give some words of encouragement, some support, the offer of a listening ear.

Talk to the person at work who looks like they might be having symptoms and say 'hey, have you thought it might be this?'

Remember that phone call with my cousin I talked about at the beginning of the book, when I had no idea what was wrong with me? That conversation was transformative. It set off a whole chain of events that led me to a diagnosis, that led me to proper treatment, that gave me my life and my happiness back.

We need to keep talking, but we need to keep listening, too.

BE LOUD

You are now in possession of the full facts, so if you hear the same old myths being peddled, challenge them. Set the record straight. Offer an educated viewpoint, give people the facts, the stats, the information they need to make an informed decision for themselves.

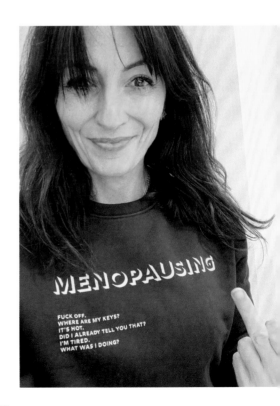

AND ABOVE ALL, BE PROUD!

You are a badass bitch.
We are ALL badass bitches.

Fuck you, menopause!

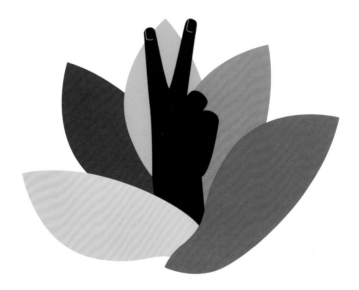

We are NOT going quietly.

MENOPAUSE WARRIORS

Dr Naomi Potter
Insta: @drmenopausecare
Naomi is SO brilliant and practical, she's the
greatest at explaining. Join her Instagram lives.

Carolyn Harris MP
Twitter: @carolynharris24
I literally LOVE Carolyn. Women like her change
the world. We need to support her, because she
changes the law for us women.

Caroline Hirons
Insta: @carolinehirons
Camouflage queen. No-bullshit skincare advice.

Diane Danzebrink
Twitter: @Dianedanz #makemenopausematter
An absolute trailblazer and founder of the
campaign that is calling for all GPs to receive
mandatory menopause training, and for a
module to be taught at every medical school.

Gabby Logan
Twitter: @GabbyLogan
Middle-aged and unashamed, you *have*
to listen to her podcast, the Mid•Point.

Dr Nighat Arif
Insta: @drnighatarif
TikTok: @drnighatarif
NHS GP and busiest woman. Tirelessly helping all
women, but especially those in her community.

Mariella Frostrup
Twitter: @mariellaf1
Journalist, campaigner and author, Mariella Frostrup
is the OG menopause warrior for me. She was the
first that I saw speak about the menopause in the
public domain. Mariella, thank you SO much. You
are an absolute woman of women.

Karen Arthur
Insta: @thekarenarthur #wearyourhappy
You might remember Karen from my documentary
– sassy, ballsy and the host of the brilliant podcast
Menopause Whilst Black.

Kate Muir
Twitter: @muirkate
Writer, activist, documentary maker and ally who
is lifting the lid on menopause, and my mate.

Samantha Evans
Insta: @samtalkssex
Our resident menopausing sexpert – what
she doesn't know isn't worth knowing.

Cathy Proctor
Insta: @meandmyhrt
Love Cathy – she really struggled finding the
right HRT combo, her Insta helps so many.

Meg Matthews
Insta: @megsmenopause
Meg uses her platform to educate people and
empower women. She is one of the Meno OGs.

Dr Anne Henderson
Insta: @gynaeexpert
Gynaecologist and British Menopause
Society-accredited specialist.

Tim Spector
Insta: @timspector
An epidemiologist, who writes about metabolism
and sugar at menopause.

Black Women in Menopause UK
Insta: @blackwomeninmenopause
Events, peer support and space to share
experiences… watch out for cool events.

Paulina Porizkova
Insta: @paulinaporizkov
Supermodel, actress, writer. Love her.

Liz Earle
Insta: @lizearleme
Midlife wellbeing expert and total legend.

Lorraine Candy
Insta: @lorrainecandy
Journalist and *Sunday Times* bestselling author.
Badass... Does an amazing podcast (see below).

Postcards from Midlife
Insta: @postcardsfrommidlife
Podcast from Lorraine Candy and Trish Halpin.

Lisa Snowdon
Insta: @lisa_snowdon
Does fantastic Instagram lives with Dr Naomi.

Dr Shahzadi Harper
Insta: @drshahzadiharper
The Perimenopause Doctor and esteemed
author of *The Perimenopause Solution*.

Jennifer Kennedy
Insta: @catastrophegalloping
Author of *Galloping Catastrophe: Musings of a
Menopausal Woman* – this woman is hilarious.

Meera Bhogal
Insta: @meerabhogal
Advice on eating well during menopause.

Buck Angel
Insta: @buckangel
He is great – a 'man with a female past, LGBTQ
innovator, plant medicine activist, tranpa'.

Tania Glyde
Insta: @queermenopause
Promotes inclusive menopause resources
and education for therapists and healthcare
practitioners about the needs of LGBTQIA+.

Jane Anne James
Insta: @janemhdg
Founder of Menopause and HRT discussion
group on Facebook. This group is lovely.

Nigel Denby
Insta: @Harleystreetathomemenopause
Specialist menopause dietitian – really very good.

MPowered Women
Insta: @mpowered_women
Experts and brilliant women to power you into
midlife. They are way ahead of the curve.

Luinluland
Insta: @luinluland
Menopause-mindset-shifter, fearless positivity
rebel and founder of the Zero Fucks Club.

Anita Powell
Insta: @blkmenobeyond
Community radio presenter, podcaster of *Black
Menopause and Beyond* and community worker.

Hormone Health
Insta: @hormonehealthuk
Private women's health clinic, founded by
Nick Panay who is the UK menopause guru.

The Latte Lounge
Insta: @loungethelatte
Online community for midlife women.

Menopausemandate
Insta: @menopausemandate
Brings together all Meno groups to get the
government to improve care. A thunderclap.

Dr Louise Newson
Insta: @menopause_doctor
Menopause specialist and all-round guru.

Lorraine Kelly
Insta: @lorrainekellysmith
No intro needed ...

INDEX

THANK YOU

DAVINA

Oh my goodness so where do I start? There have been so many women and men that have been part of my menopausing journey. I would like to start by thanking all the menopause warriors out there. Tirelessly tapping away on social media via blogs reels tweets ... anything to try and help women navigate midlife and our second spring. You are a source of great comfort and I have loved every minute of tweeting away together in the evenings, so thank you. You know who you are and many of you've been name checked in the back of this book.

I also want to give special love to Kat Keogh, for organising me and helping me to focus (quite a tricky task) and being such a menopause font of all knowledge. HQ, thank you for existing, and Lisa Milton you have made all this possible. Thank you from the bottom of my heart. Thank you to my brilliant designers, Imagist, and wonderful photographer Mark Hayman.

And also to Louise McKeever from HQ. OMG!!!!! Thank you for all your patience and thank you so much for "getting" me. You really, really are brilliant. Thank you to Amanda Harris. You know how much I love you. I could never have done this without you.

Also, to Emily and Molly, my agents and friends. I feel very blessed having you both in my life. Georgie White, nobody would know anything about menopausing if you didn't help me get it out there. Thank you for nudging me onto Tik Tok ...

A huge thank you to Dr Naomi Potter. I fell in love with Naomi via Instagram. She is forensic in her delivery of information. And takes amazing care to make sure it is easy to understand and digest. She does such great work getting the message out there to us all. I have deep respect and admiration for you x

A huge heartfelt debt of gratitude to all the women that sent us their sometimes heart-breaking, sometimes uplifting, menopausing stories. Your stories will help other women not feel so alone. And as we know, it can feel like a very lonely, isolating time.

Thank you to our contributors. Caroline Hirons (a fantastic part of our HQ fam), Cheryl Phelps-Gardiner (love) and Michael Douglas, who deserves a special mention. Thank you, Michael, for being so wise. You are my sounding board. And I value and respect you so much.

And finally Holly, Tilly and Chester. Sorry mummy was bonkers.

DR NAOMI

Thank you to Mike, my parents Carol and Ron, Jacob, Ben, Ollie, Rosie and Isla for being there always. Thank you also to Dr Kate Lethaby and Dr Alison Macbeth for their last minute, speedy and thorough eye casting which was most appreciated. Of course, finally, thank you to Davina for her boundless passion and enthusiasm without which this book would not be written and many women would still be suffering in silence.